POCKET SURGERY

POCKET NOTEBOOK

POCKET SURGERY

Edited by

Paul J. Mosca, M.D., Ph.D.
Assistant Research Professor
Chief Resident
Department of General and Thoracic Surgery
Duke University Medical Center
Durham, North Carolina

Lisa A. Clark, M.D.
Assistant Professor of Surgery, Division of General Surgery
Durham Regional Hospital
Department of General and Thoracic Surgery
Duke University Medical Center
Durham, North Carolina

H. Kim Lyerly, M.D., F.A.C.S.
Professor of Surgery, Division of General Surgery
Director, Program in Molecular Therapeutics
Department of General and Thoracic Surgery
Duke University Medical Center
Durham, North Carolina

Theodore N. Pappas, M.D., F.A.C.S.
Professor of Surgery, Division of General Surgery
Director, Residency Program in General and Thoracic Surgery
Department of General and Thoracic Surgery
Duke University Medical Center
Chief of Surgery, Durham VA Medical Center
Durham, North Carolina

LIPPINCOTT WILLIAMS & WILKINS
A Wolters Kluwer Company
Philadelphia • Baltimore • New York • London
Buenos Aires • Hong Kong • Sydney • Tokyo

Acquisitions Editor: Lisa McAllister
Developmental Editor: Gina Gerace
Production Editor: Emmeline A. Parker
Cover Designer: Patricia Gast
Compositor: Keithley and Associates, Inc.
Printer: Victor Graphics

530 Walnut Street
Philadelphia, PA 19106 USA
LWW.com

Printed in the USA

Library of Congress Cataloging-in-Publication Data

Pocket surgery / Paul J. Mosca ... [et al.].
p. ; cm. — (Pocket notebook)
Includes bibliographical references and index.
ISBN 0-7817-3579-3
1. Surgery—Handbooks, manuals, etc. 2. Surgery, Operative—Handbooks, manuals, etc.
I. Mosca, Paul J. II. Series.
[DNLM: 1. Surgical Procedures, Operative—Handbooks. WO 39 P7394 2001]
RD37.P63 2001
617'.91—dc21

2001045078

Care has been taken to confirm the accuracy of the information presented and to describe generally accepted practices. However, the authors, editors, and publisher are not responsible for errors or omissions or for any consequences from application of the information in this book and make no warranty, expressed or implied, with respect to the currency, completeness, or accuracy of the contents of the publication. Application of this information in a particular situation remains the professional responsibility of the practitioner.

The authors, editors, and publisher have exerted every effort to ensure that drug selection and dosage set forth in this text are in accordance with current recommendations and practice at the time of publication. However, in view of ongoing research, changes in government regulations, and the constant flow of information relating to drug therapy and drug reactions, the reader is urged to check the package insert for each drug for any change in indications and dosage and for added warnings and precautions. This is particularly important when the recommended agent is a new or infrequently employed drug.

Some drugs and medical devices presented in this publication have Food and Drug Administration (FDA) clearance for limited use in restricted research settings. It is the responsibility of the health care provider to ascertain the FDA status of each drug or device planned for use in their clinical practice.

10 9 8 7 6 5 4 3 2 1

My contribution to this work is dedicated to my lovely wife Kathy, our sons Jimmy, Matthew, and Neil, and my parents, Carlo and Dorinda.

Paul Mosca

My gratitude to Walt Pickett, Jim and Mindy Elliott, and Al and Linda Clark.

Lisa Clark

I express my thanks to the housestaff and their families.

Kim Lyerly

This handbook is dedicated to our mentors, Dr. David C. Sabiston, Jr., and Dr. Robert W. Anderson.

Ted Pappas

Contents

Contributing Authors

Thomas A. Aloia, M.D.
Senior Assistant Resident
Department of General and Thoracic Surgery
Duke University Medical Center
Durham, North Carolina

Lisa A. Clark, M.D.
Assistant Professor of Surgery, Division of General Surgery
Durham Regional Hospital
Department of General and Thoracic Surgery
Duke University Medical Center
Durham, North Carolina

Pierre DeMatos, M.D.
Attending Surgeon
Regional Surgical Specialists
Asheville, North Carolina

Patrick W. Domkowski, M.D., Ph.D.
Senior Assistant Resident
Department of General and Thoracic Surgery
Duke University Medical Center
Durham, North Carolina

Sitaram M. Emani, M.D.
Senior Assistant Resident
Department of General and Thoracic Surgery
Duke University Medical Center
Durham, North Carolina

G. V. Gonzalez-Stawinski, M.D.
Senior Assistant Resident
Department of General and Thoracic Surgery
Duke University Medical Center
Durham, North Carolina

M. Todd Jacobs, M.D.
Fellow in Musculoskeletal Radiology
Department of Radiology
Duke University Medical Center
Durham, North Carolina

H. Kim Lyerly, M.D., F.A.C.S.
Professor of Surgery, Division of General Surgery
Associate Professor of Pathology
Assistant Professor of Immunology
Director, Program in Molecular Therapeutics
Department of General and Thoracic Surgery
Duke University Medical Center
Durham, North Carolina

Samuel M. Mahaffey, M.D., M.B.A.
Associate Professor of Surgery in Pediatrics
Medical Director, Perioperative Services
Department of General and Thoracic Surgery
Duke University Medical Center
Durham, North Carolina

Paul J. Mosca, M.D., Ph.D.
Assistant Research Professor
Chief Resident
Department of General and Thoracic Surgery
Duke University Medical Center
Durham, North Carolina

Mark W. Onaitis, M.D.
Senior Assistant Resident
Department of General and Thoracic Surgery
Duke University Medical Center
Durham, North Carolina

Theodore N. Pappas, M.D., F.A.C.S.
Professor of Surgery, Division of General Surgery
Director, Residency Program in General and Thoracic Surgery
Department of General and Thoracic Surgery
Duke University Medical Center
Chief of Surgery, Durham VA Medical Center
Durham, North Carolina

G. Robert Stephenson, Jr., M.D.
Senior Assistant Resident
Department of General and Thoracic Surgery
Duke University Medical Center
Durham, North Carolina

Bryan C. Weidner, M.D.
Senior Fellow, Division of Pediatric Surgery
Department of Surgery
Children's Hospital and Medical Center
University of Washington School of Medicine
Seattle, Washington

David C. White, M.D.
Senior Assistant Resident
Department of General and Thoracic Surgery
Duke University Medical Center
Durham, North Carolina

Rebekah R. White, M.D.
Senior Assistant Resident
Howard Hughes Postdoctoral Research Fellow
Department of General and Thoracic Surgery
Duke University Medical Center
Durham, North Carolina

Preface

A unique aspect of surgical residency that is challenging to even the brightest and most gifted of graduating medical students is the process of learning an enormous body of knowledge while developing good judgment and technical prowess in surgery. Numerous learning aids are available to assist with this task, but there is no replacement for diligent work, long hours in the hospital, and training under dedicated educators and role models. This handbook is *not a substitute* for extensive reading or for any aspect of traditional surgical training. Instead, it is designed to *remind and reinforce*, and the editors hope that it will facilitate an early mastery of the operative and perioperative management of surgical patients.

The purpose of this manual is to provide easily portable, key information to residents or students for use during day-to-day patient care. It contains a convenient, alphabetically organized section of brief synopses reviewing the basic steps of common surgical procedures. In addition, the *Pocket Notebook* contains a variety of easily referenced tables for organizing personal and valuable information.

Disclaimer: It would be impossible to encapsulate all common operative procedures or all potential variations in operative and perioperative management in a single pocket-sized handbook; we therefore made no attempt to do so. This book does not represent a standard of care or practice guideline, and under no circumstances should it be construed as such.

Although it is hoped that this version of *Pocket Surgery* is as helpful to residents and medical students as the authors intend, readers are encouraged to offer suggestions regarding potential improvements in the handbook. Comments may be e-mailed to Paul Mosca at *pjm65@duke.edu*.

POCKET SURGERY

Chapter I

GENERAL INFORMATION

Section 1: Personal Data

Name: ______________________________

Phone #: ______________________________

Pager #: ______________________________

Cell-phone #: ______________________________

Address: ______________________________

____

____

Section 2: Hospital Information

HOSPITAL # 1:		
Dictation #s		
Computer Codes		
Copier Codes		
Other #s		

HOSPITAL # 2:		
Dictation #s		
Computer Codes		
Copier Codes		
Other #s		

HOSPITAL # 3:		
Dictation #s		
Computer Codes		
Copier Codes		
Other #s		

Key phone numbers: **HOSPITAL # 1:**		
Location	**Phone # 1**	**Phone # 2**
ER		
Radiology:		
Body CT		
Neuro CT		
MRI		
Ultrasound		
Vascular Radiology		
Neuroradiology		
Labs:		
Chemistry		
Hematology		
Microbiology		
Blood gas		
Coagulation		
Serology		
Cardiology Studies:		
Echo		
Funct Studies		

Key phone numbers: **HOSPITAL # 2:**		
Location	**Phone # 1**	**Phone # 2**
ER		
Radiology:		
Body CT		
Neuro CT		
MRI		
Ultrasound		
Vascular Radiology		
Neuroradiology		
Labs:		
Chemistry		
Hematology		
Microbiology		
Blood gas		
Coagulation		
Serology		
Cardiology Studies:		
Echo		
Funct Studies		

Key phone numbers: **HOSPITAL # 3:**		
Location	**Phone # 1**	**Phone # 2**
ER		
Radiology:		
Body CT		
Neuro CT		
MRI		
Ultrasound		
Vascular Radiology		
Neuroradiology		
Labs:		
Chemistry		
Hematology		
Microbiology		
Blood gas		
Coagulation		
Serology		
Cardiology Studies:		
Echo		
Funct Studies		

OTHER PHONE NUMBERS:		
Name/Location	**Phone # 1**	**Phone # 2**

Chapter II

Perioperative Care of the Surgical Patient

Preoperative Preparation

Perioperative care of the surgical patient encompasses preoperative preparation, operative management, and postoperative care. Each interval has important caveats that emphasize specific elements of patient care. General preoperative preparation should include an overall assessment of the patient, consisting of a thorough history and physical examination. Once a diagnosis and the need for an operation have been established, it is critical that the patient's physiologic status be optimized to the extent possible during the preoperative period in order to minimize perioperative morbidity and mortality. This is usually feasible for elective cases. However, in the case of urgent procedures, circumstances may allow only enough time for rapid correction of volume, hemodynamic and electrolyte abnormalities and possibly glucose control. In emergency cases, it may be necessary to complete resuscitation in the operating room.

The **risk factors** for the major systems are:

Pulmonary/Respiratory: > 20 pack/yr smoking history (smoking cessation eight weeks prior to surgery reduces pulmonary complications), COPD ($pO_2 < 60$ mmHg or $pCO_2 > 50$ mmHg), or recent abdominal or thoracic surgery

Cardiac: Congestive heart failure (CHF), Coronary artery disease (CAD) or dysrhythmias

Vascular: Severe hypertension (DBP > 110 mmHg, usually previously untreated) or peripheral vascular disease

Renal: Renal insufficiency (BUN > 50 mg/dl or creatinine > 3.0 mg/dl) or acute renal failure

Endocrine: Diabetes mellitus (Type I and II), chronic steroid use

Hematologic: Leukopenia, thrombocytopenia, disseminated intravascular coagulopathy (DIC)

In addition, the patient must be fully aware of the risks and benefits of surgery (see Chapter III). For both medical and legal reasons, an informed consent is signed by the patient prior to surgery and only after a conversation between the patient and the surgeon. Many hospitals require the presence and signature of a witness (healthcare provider not involved in the surgery) during consent. This protects both the patient and the doctor.

Specific ordering of preoperative labs and other tests (e.g., EKG, chest x-ray) will depend on the planned procedure and will vary with each institution, surgeon and anesthesiologist. *All* patients should have a thorough history and physical examination. In general, an EKG is warranted for patients older than 40 years of age or with a personal or family history of heart disease. Similarly, a PA/LAT chest film is needed only if the patient is ≥ 40, has a history of pulmonary disease (e.g. COPD or emphysema), or a thoracic procedure is planned. Laboratory tests (e.g., CBC, electrolytes, PT/PTT, and type and screen or type and cross) are tailored to the patient and procedure. For many ambulatory general surgery procedures (e.g., inguinal herniorraphy) a complete blood count, basic serum chemistries (Na^+, K^+, Cl^-, CO_2, BUN, creatinine and glucose), and urinalysis, in addition to the H&P, may be entirely adequate. For larger procedures (e.g., colon resection or vascular procedure), it is necessary to have, in addition the aforementioned labs, a PT/PTT, T/S and T/C.

General Considerations

For elective cases patients are made NPO after midnight except for necessary oral medications with sips of water. As many patients are at home the night before their elective surgery, they are instructed not to eat after midnight. If intravenous fluids or medications are needed prior to surgery, then these patients are generally admitted the night before the operation. In the case of elective bowel procedures, bowel preparation can again take place either at home or in the hospital. Although the method of bowel preparation may vary widely among institutions and attendings, there are two fundamental components. First, the ***mechanical***: the bowel contents are evacuated and this is typically accomplished with a combination of taking PO laxatives (e.g., polyethylene glycol, magnesium citrate) ± enemas. Second, the ***antimicrobial***: bacterial counts of the colon are decreased by administering an enteral, non-absorbable antibiotic such as neomycin. Once the patient is in the operating room, gastric decompression (NGT/OGT) and insertion of a foley urinary catheter may be indicated. For patient comfort this should be performed once the patient is asleep. Skin preparation should include a shower the night prior to surgery with a topical antibacterial agent such as hibiclens. In addition, if hair must be removed from the surgical site, it ideally should be ***clipped***, not shaved, ***just prior to*** *surgery* (for example, in the preoperative holding area). Thromboembolic prophylaxis such as venous compression stockings and/or **sequential compression boots** should be placed ***prior to*** *surgery*.

Preoperative management of the diabetic patient requires special consideration. Oral hypoglycemic agents should be discontinued 1 day prior to elective surgery. For patients dependent on insulin, **one-half of the normal dose** should be administered on the morning of surgery. It will also be necessary to check the patient's **blood glucose level** prior to surgery and provide **glucose-containing IV fluids** at an appropriate rate.

Patients taking coumadin and at continued high risk for thrombosis must have procedures performed through a **heparin window**. For unfractionated heparin, patients discontinue coumadin about 3 days prior to surgery and are admitted the following day for administration of an IV heparin drip (titrated to a PTT of 50–70). For non-vascular procedures, unfractionated IV heparin may be discontinued approximately 6 hours prior to surgery and resumed 6–12 hours following the completion of surgery; for vascular surgery, heparin is often continued up to the time of the procedure, depending on the type of surgery. An alternative approach to the heparin drip is to instruct patients to begin self-administering therapeutic doses of low-molecular weight heparin (LMWH) at home after discontinuing coumadin; the last dose of LMWH may be administered about 24 hours prior to surgery, and it is resumed prior to restarting coumadin postoperatively. Coumadin administration is generally resumed 2–3 days following surgery. This window allows surgery to be completed while the concomitant risks of a thrombotic or embolic event are minimized.

Patients on chronic steroids prior to surgery or those with known adrenal insufficiency are typically given "**stress dose**" steroids. Typically, hydrocortisone 100 mg IV on call to OR will cover most adult patients. This may be re-dosed in the recovery room following surgery and again 8–12 hours later, or administered as a rapid taper.

Perioperative antibiotics

Antibiotics may be used either **prophylactically** or **therapeutically** (Tables II.1 and II.2, respectively) in the perioperative period. In either case, it is important that the antibiotic selected covers the most likely pathogen(s) present based on the particular surgical procedure and/or available microbiologic data. For proper prophylaxis, serum antibiotic levels must be in the therapeutic range at the **time of incision** in order to achieve the antibiotic benefit. Most intravenous antibiotics therefore should be administered 30–60 minutes prior to incision, depending upon the rate of infusion (for example, Vancomycin typically requires at least 60 minutes for infusion). Antibiotics are typically re-dosed intraoperatively if the case lasts 4 hours or longer.

In general, intravenous antibiotics should be administered for the following types of cases: clean-contaminated procedures, contaminated procedures, or dirty procedures; high-risk patients (immunosuppressed patients, those with established mitral valve prolapse or IV drug abusers), or patients with prosthetic material (e.g. mechanical heart valves, pacemakers or indwelling catheters). Although it is a common practice, data supporting intravenous antibiotic administration prophylactically routinely for most clean cases are lacking.

Table II.1. Examples of Antibiotic Prophylaxis Regimens[a] in General/Vascular Surgery[1–3]

Type of Procedure	First Line Antibiotic(s)	Alternative Antibiotic(s)
Cardiothoracic	Cefazolin or Cefuroxime[b]	Vancomycin
Gastrointestinal		
Upper	Cefazolin	Clindamycin
Liver/Pancreas/ Biliary Tract/Kidney	Cefazolin	Ciprofloxacin/Clindamycin *or* Ciprofloxacin/Metronidazole
Appendix	Cefoxitin or Cefotetan	Ciprofloxacin/Metronidazole
Colorectal	Neomycin/Erythromycin base (P.O.), in addition to mechanical bowel prep	Cefoxitin (I.V.)[c] *or* Ciprofloxacin/Metronidazole (I.V.)[c]
Head and Neck	Cefazolin	Vancomycin
Vascular	Cefazolin	Vancomycin
Other Clean Procedures (no prosthetic material)	None	
SBE Prophylaxis[d]	Ampicillin *or* Ampicillin/Gentamicin (latter for high-risk or GI procedures)	Vancomycin *or* Vancomycin/Gentamicin (latter for high-risk or GI procedures)

[a] Typically administered preoperatively up to 24 hours postoperatively.

[b] IV abx may be continued until thoracostomy tubes are removed.

[c] Often given in addition to standard bowel preparation, though not of proven benefit based on published literature.

[d] One hour preoperatively and up to 24 hours postoperatively.

Table II.2. Examples of Initial/Empiric Antibiotic Treatment in General and Vascular Surgery Infections in the Absence of Microbiologic Data

Type of Procedure	First Line Antibiotic(s)	Alternative Antibiotic(s)
Cardiothoracic (e.g., empyema)	Cefazolin	Vancomycin
Gastrointestinal		
Upper	Ampicillin/Sulbactam	Ciprofloxacin/Metronidazole
Liver/Pancreas/ Biliary Tract/Kidney	Ampicillin/Sulbactam	Ciprofloxacin/Metronidazole
Appendix	Ampicillin/Sulbactam	Ciprofloxacin/Metronidazole
Colorectal (bowel prep not possible)	Ampicillin/Sulbactam	Ciprofloxacin/Metronidazole
Head and Neck	Cefazolin	Vancomycin
Vascular		
Graft infection	Cefazolin	Vancomycin
Diabetic foot infection or gangrene	Ticarcillin/Clavulanate *or* Piperacillin/Tazobactam	e.g., Imipenem *or* Ciprofloxacin/Clindamycin

Postoperative Care

Any general or vascular surgery procedure in which the patient returns to the ward requires a standard set of guidelines for proper and thorough care. The patient must be approached systematically so that nothing is overlooked. Close attention to the patient's level of conscious and adequacy of pain control is vital. Objective signs regarding pain control are usually increased heart rate and/or blood pressure. One should also carefully assess oxygen saturation, urine and drain output, the physical examination, and other relevant data.

Respiratory: The otherwise healthy patient should have normal respirations (12–18/minute) and have oxygen saturation above 95%. If feasible, it is beneficial to elevate the head of the bed to 30°. This utilizes gravity to provide a mechanical advantage for diaphragmatic excursion, thus increasing tidal volumes, and allows oral secretions to be cleared more easily. It is also important to monitor not only the number of respirations, but also the quality. Short shallow breaths may indicate increased pain, premature extubation from surgery, or a pneumothorax. Breath sounds should be auscultated and a CXR obtained if indicated. Respirations may improve with elevating the head of the bed (unless contraindicated), incentive spirometry, and providing oxygen by nasal cannula or face mask if necessary. If severe respiratory distress occurs postoperatively, the clinician should also obtain an ABG, as well as an EKG in patients with elevated cardiac risk, and should have a low threshold for re-intubation. Narcotic overdose, pulmonary edema, myocardial infarction, and pulmonary embolus should always be included in the differential diagnosis. The causes for severe respiratory distress are numerous and should be assessed in an environment in which the airway is properly controlled.

Cardiovascular: Both the rate and rhythm require monitoring postoperatively. Tachycardia is usually indicative of hypovolemia or inadequate pain control, the former typically being associated with a normal or low BP and the latter with hypertension. A critical point to remember is that ***postoperative hypotension and/or tachycardia should be assumed to reflect hemorrhage until proven otherwise***. In healthy patients with normal renal function, urine output (acceptable for adults being > 0.5 cc/kg/hr) is very helpful in the assessment of volume status. Because of "third-spacing" of fluid associated with surgical stress, a variable amount of additional volume replacement with crystalloid solution is to be expected in order to achieve intravascular volume repletion. Assessing skin temperature and capillary refill in the extremities, as well as the peripheral pulses, is helpful in assessing the adequacy of tissue perfusion. Hypothermia should be avoided, as this may increase cardiac complications and, if severe, is associated with postoperative coagulopathy.

Renal: Urine output in the patient with normal renal function typically reflects intravascular volume status and adequacy of tissue perfusion. Monitoring the BUN, creatinine, and BUN/creatinine ratio may also be helpful in selected patients and may complement data regarding urine output. For patients with postoperative oliguria, calculating the fractional excretion of sodium (FENa) may be informative:

[(Urine NA) (Serum creatinine) / (Urine creatinine) (Serum sodium)] X 100

If the FENa is < 1 %, it indicates pre-renal azotemia (usually associated with intravascular volume depletion, but also consistent with heart failure). If the FENa > 2 %, it suggests intrinsic renal parenchymal dysfunction. Urine sodium is also helpful in assessing volume status in the patient with normal renal function. A urine sodium of < 20 suggests pre-renal azotemia, whereas a urine sodium > 40 indicates intrinsic renal dysfunction.

Gastrointestinal: Following a major abdominal procedure in which a postoperative ileus is expected, the patient is intially NPO, and sometimes a NGT is placed and kept to continuous low suction for a brief period. After there is evidence of bowel function, such as with the passage of flatus (typically postoperative day 2–5, depending on the procedure), the patient may be able to take clears or a soft diet and is advanced as tolerated to the appropriate postoperative diet. A patient who is effectively without nutrition for 7–10 days perioperatively requires postoperative enteral tube feeds (e.g., via a feeding jejunostomy tube or nasoduodenal tube), or, if enteral feeds are not feasible, total parenteral nutrition.

Endocrine: In the diabetic patient, particular attention should be given to glucose control, which can be checked in the postoperative recovery unit, on arrival to the ward, and every 6 hours (or qac + qhs) thereafter. In addition to an appropriate basal insulin dose, the patient should have an insulin sliding scale as a part of the routine postoperative orders: *For example,* for

Glucose	0–60	Give juice and/or 1/2 – 1 amp D_{50}, call house officer
	61–200	No additional insulin
	201–250	2 units regular insulin sq
	251–300	4 units regular insulin sq
	301–350	6 units regular insulin sq
	351–400	8 units regular insulin sq
	> 400	10 units regular insulin sq, call house officer

Until adequate POs are taken, glucose-containing IV fluids are often provided. Once normal PO intake has resumed following the operation the patient should return to the normal preoperative insulin regimen. For those patients on steroids prior to surgery or those with adrenal insufficiency, perioperative stress dose steroids, or a rapid steroid taper, are often administered (controversial); an example is hydrocortisone 100 mg IV on induction and q8 hours to a total of 3 doses.

Wound care: It is critical that the surgeon examine the wound **every day** postoperatively and assess for signs of erythema, induration or drainage. The proper healing wound should have a healing ridge and be dry and non-erythematous. Drainage may represent a superficial wound infection or possible dehiscence, or may simply reflect fat necrosis. The appearance and odor of the drainage should be assessed as well as the overall clinical picture (e.g., fever, white count). Excessive tension on the wound, foreign material, hematomas, malnutrition, poor tissue oxygenation, infection, diabetes, obesity and chronic steroid use are among factors that impede wound healing.

Chapter III

OPERATIVE PROCEDURES

General Considerations

Indications: Consider degree of urgency — ***Emergent vs Urgent vs Elective***. When possible, in seriously ill patients, aggressive resuscitation and application of temporizing interventions (e.g., percutaneous drainage of fluid collections) may convert surgical emergencies into urgencies, and urgencies into elective procedures (or sometimes nonoperative therapy).

Setup: For *all* procedures,

1. Resuscitation, stabilization and preoperative preparation are the first priorities
2. Imaging studies or other aids should be placed within view from the OR table
3. Pt must be positioned appropriately
4. Consider whether NGT/OGT, Foley, SCDs are indicated
5. Consider whether IV Abx, stress-dose steroids are indicated
6. Consider donning and adjusting headlight, surgical loupes; ALWAYS wear appropriate eye protection
7. Always have operative plan in mind before starting procedure

Procedure:

1. Make **incision** so as **to optimize exposure**
2. Remember to **explore** abdomen when appropriate at the start of a procedure
3. In taking down **adhesions**, remember to do what's easy first, go from known to unknown, divide only translucent avascular planes when possible, avoid unnecessary dissection, and, if you are not making progress, try something else
4. Ensure **proper exposure** using appropriate retractors, and reassess exposure if you are struggling
5. During closure of fascia, consider placing **retention sutures/spoons** in setting of impaired wound healing (e.g., immunosuppression, malnutrition, infection)
6. In setting of intra-abdominal infection or gross soilage, **avoid primary closure** of skin, such as by packing wound and allowing healing by secondary intention, using delayed primary closure (packing initially, and reapproximating skin edges in 3–4 days), or by placing widely spaced staples or sutures and "wicking"

Postop: In every pt, postoperative hemodynamic instability, tachycardia and/or oliguria must be assumed due to hypovolemia/bleeding until proven otherwise

Risks: The following is a list of **general perioperative risks/complications** that may occur with a wide variety of surgical procedures: Hemorrhage, infection, wound dehiscence ± evisceration, injury to organs, MI, stroke, pneumonia, ileus, bowel obstruction, urinary retention, DVT/PE; death

Section 1
General/Transplant Surgery

Adrenalectomy — Open, Anterior Approach: Left Side (Right in *italics*) [4]

Indications:

Adrenal adenoma, pheochromocytoma, adrenocortical carcinoma, selected incidentalomas or metastatic tumors; rarely, bilateral adrenalectomy for adrenal hyperplasia refractory to medical Tx or after failed hypophysectomy in selected pts

Preop/Setup:

Pheo: Alpha adrenergic blockade 5–7 days preop, then beta blockade if tachycardic, volume repletion if needed
Aldosteronoma: K+ repletion
Cushing's/adrenal adenoma: steroid prep
Position = Supine; arterial line & central venous monitoring (± Swan) often indicated; Foley, NGT; SCDs

Procedure:

1. Left (*right*) subcostal/hockey-stick, bilat. subcostal, or midline **incision**
2. **Explore** abd. for extra-adrenal (esp. peri-aortic)/contralat. pheo., metastatic dz, etc.
3. Place self-retaining **retractor** with moist lap pads protecting viscera
4. Retract splenic flexure (*hepatic flexure*) of colon inferiorly, **enter lesser sac** through gastrocolic ligament
5. **Expose:** incise peritoneum & anterior Gerota's fascia and reflect pancreas superiorly, or (alt) mobilize spleen & pancreatic tail medially (*Kocherize duodenum, mobilize liver superiorly by dividing inferolateral peritoneal attachments*)
6. **Identify**: Left adrenal gland & superior pole of kidney (*right adrenal gland, superior pole of kidney, IVC*)
7. **Alert** anesthesia of potential for profound hypertension (catecholamine release) or hypotension (cessation of catecholamine release) as adrenal dissection is undertaken
8. Begin **dissection** of adrenal laterally and work medially, clipping, ligating and/or electrocauterizing vessels
9. **Ligate** adrenal **vein** before arteries and as early as possible for pheochromocytoma to diminish release of catecholamines into systemic circ. (*note: placement of right angle or side biting clamp on IVC may be needed for ligation/division of right adrenal vein*)
10. Complete dissection and remove adrenal gland, **close** abdominal wall, fascia, & skin

Postop: In immediate postop period, monitor hemodynamics/volume status, electrolyte disturbances, potential for adrenal crisis

Risks: Hemorrhage/hematoma, life-threatening hemodynamic changes, acute adrenal insufficiency, injury to organs (e.g., kidney, pancreas, liver, duodenum), wound or intra-abdominal infection, pancreatitis, pleural effusion, failure to cure disease (incorrect localization or dx, or failure to eradicate disease [e.g., extra-adrenal or bilateral pheochromocytoma, metastatic or residual tumor, etc.])

Adrenalectomy — Laparoscopic, Transabdomial: Left Side (Right in *italics*) [5,6]

Indications: Similar to open, except see contraindications

Contraindications:

***Absolute*:** Uncorrectable coagulopathy; inadequate surgical skill or equipment; inability of pt to tolerate general anesthesia or pneumoperitoneum
***Relative*:** Multiple prior abdominal operations/dense adhesions (use open or retroperitoneal approach); primary malignancy, especially with significant local invasion; extra-adrenal disease; presence of diaphragmatic hernia

Setup:

Position = Supine, ipsilat side (to pathology) elevated 30–45° (or alt right [*left*] lat decubitus, table bent [convex] at waist), reverse T-berg; a-line & central venous monitoring (± Swan) often indicated; NGT/OGT; SCDs; 30° scope

Procedure:

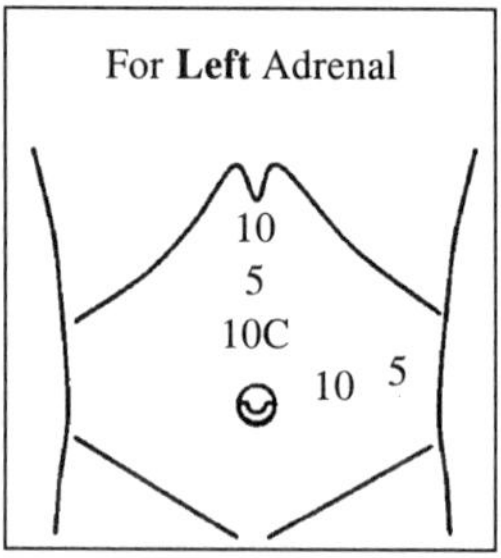

1. **Ports**: camera (10 mm [10C]) trocar ~ 1/2 to 2/3 dist. from xiphoid to umbilicus, liver retractor (10 mm) trocar subxiphoid, optional assistant (5 mm) trocar between these, surgeon's dominant hand (10 mm) & nondominant/ retracting hand (5 mm) trocars ~ level of umbilicus on ipsilat side
2. **Explore** abd (metastatic dz, contralat. or extra-adrenal pheo)
3. **Expose**: Mobilize prox. descending colon, splenocolic & splenorenal ligaments, lateral splenic attachments, let spleen fall medially (*mobilize hepatic flexure, retroperitoneal attachments of liver*); consider ultrasonic dissector
4. **Identify**: Left adrenal gland & superior pole of kidney (*right adrenal gland, superior pole of kidney, duodenum, IVC*)
5. **Open** Gerota's fascia, carefully retract kidney inferiorly (*and liver superiorly*)
6. **Alert** anesthesia of potential for profound hypertension (catecholamine release) or hypotension (cessation of catecholamine release) as adrenal dissection is undertaken
7. **Dissect** lateral aspect of adrenal gland, then inferior where main left adrenal vein (which joins renal v.) is identified, clipped/ligated and divided (*Rt. side:expose and ligate/divide adrenal v. entering IVC; cont. dissection superiorly)*

8. **Complete** dissection of adrenal, medial to lateral, inferior to superior fashion (while minimizing direct manipulation of gland)
9. Place adrenal in plastic bag, **retrieve** through 10 mm port site, ensure hemostasis
10. **Close** port sites

Postop: See OPEN approach

Risks: Same as for open adrenalectomy, plus air embolus, trocar site hernia, and conversion to open adrenalectomy

Anal/Peri-rectal Procedures

ANAL FISTULOTOMY

Indications: Persistent symptomatic anal fistula (which generally results from an infection in an anal crypt) that does not involve the external sphincter.

Setup: Position = prone jack-knife or lithotomy, based on location of fistula

Procedure:

1. Mildly **dilate** and inspect anus/rectum
2. Gently **probe** anal crypts with fistula probe to identify fistula
3. **Cut** down on the probe, continuing to advance the probe into the fistula and cut open the fistula until the internal opening is found

Postop: Place pt on analgesics, stool softener, and sitz baths

Risks: Bleeding, fecal incontinence

HEMORRHOIDECTOMY

Indications: Symptomatic hemorrhoids that have failed medical therapy (stool softeners, sitz baths, topical treatments) or banding, bleeding, hemorrhoidal crisis

Setup: Position = prone jack-knife or lithotomy

Procedure:

1. Gently **dilate** and thoroughly examine the rectum/anus with anoscope and/or proctoscope to identify symptomatic hemorrhoids
2. Use Hill-Ferguson retractor to fully **expose** each hemorrhoid
3. Infiltrate with **local** anesthetic with epinephrine (optional if other anesthesia is administered)
4. Create triangular or elliptical **incision** to fully remove the hemorrhoid and mucosa (leaving the sphincter muscles completely intact) and oversew; alternatively, clamp hemorrhoid within Kelly, place figure-of-eight at proximal end of hemorrhoid, oversew over clamp, amputate hemorrhoid and remove clamp
5. Remove **additional** hemorrhoid(s) (up to three, but excision of all three hemorrhoidal cushions may increase risk of stricture)

Postop: Place pt on analgesics, stool softener, and sitz baths

Risks: Bleeding, fecal incontinence, recurrence, stricture

PERI-RECTAL ABSCESS DRAINAGE

Indications: Abscess around anorectum generally presenting with fullness, exquisite pain, ± fever, leukocytosis, purulent drainage

Setup: Position = Lithotomy or prone jack-knife

Procedure:

1. Examine the anus and rectum for evidence of abscess, fistula, mass, or inflammatory bowel disease with **anoscopy/proctoscopy**
2. **Anesthetize** affected area with lidocaine (if not using spinal/general anesthesia)
3. **Open** abscess cavity widely by making radially oriented incision and spreading with Kelly clamp, drain pus, examine cavity (digitally, if large) and break up loculations
4. Copiously **irrigate** wound
5. **Consider** placement of small (12–14 F) dePezzer/mushroom-tip catheter (with extra fenestrations cut in tip); alternatively, may pack with ribbon gauze

Post-op: Analgesics, stool softeners, sitz baths, care to keep incision open to allow healing from the base up (with indwelling catheter, or with wound packing)

Risks: Bleeding, fecal incontinence, recurrence of abscess, sepsis, fistula

Appendectomy — Open [4]

Indications:

Emergent: Generalized peritonitis/acute perforation (rebound, guarding)
Urgent: Suspected acute appendicitis with localized peritoneal signs (RLQ rebound tenderness, guarding, +psoas sign, +obturator sign, pain/mass on digital rectal exam)
Semi-elective: Interval appendectomy — 6 weeks after walled-off perforation treated by percutaneous drainage + abx

Setup: Position = supine

Procedure:

1. Transverse (Rocky-Davis) or oblique (McBurney's) **incision** over site of maximal tenderness; attempt to remain lateral to rectus sheath if possible
2. Bluntly spread (perpendicularly) through abdominal muscle layers, sharply through fasciae to find peritoneum and **enter** peritoneal cavity; consider culturing peritoneal fluid if turbid
3. **Locate** cecum and find base of appendix at convergence of teniae coli, **deliver** appendix into wound, **assess** whether inflamed, purulent, gangrenous, perforated
4. *Regardless* of whether appendix is inflamed, ligate and divide **mesoappendix** in continuity working from tip to base (2-0 or 3-0 absorbable ligatures)
5. Place 3-0 silk/vicryl **pursestring** (or "Z" stitch) suture in cecum around appendiceal base
6. **Clamp** appendix at base to crush, then reclamp just distally, doubly ligate appendix between this clamp & cecum with 0 chromic gut; excise appendix with electrocautery or scalpel, pass contaminated knife off field [cauterizing stump controversial]
7. **Invert** appendiceal stump into cecum with forceps as pursestring (or "Z" stitch) is tightened
8. Inspect RLQ peritoneal cavity for abscess; copiously **irrigate** with saline; drain RLQ if abscess present
9. If appendix is not grossly inflamed, **R/O** Crohn's, diverticulitis, Meckel's diverticulitis, GYN pathol. in women, perf'd. gastric or duodenal ulcer, cholecystitis (may need larger/2nd incision)
10. **Close** abdomen in layers with absorbable suture; staple skin or use subcuticular closure/steri-strips; close muscle but leave skin and subcutaneous tissue open for secondary intention or delayed primary closure 3–5 days later if significant peritoneal contamination present

Risks: Hemorrhage, bowel injury, ileus, abscess, SBO, wound infection, infertility (women) in setting of perforation

Appendectomy — Laparoscopic [7]

Indications: Same as for open; may be preferred if diagnosis uncertain (i.e. woman of childbearing age) or in obese patients

Setup: Position = supine or modified lithotomy with slight Trendelenberg; Foley, consider NGT/OGT

Procedure:

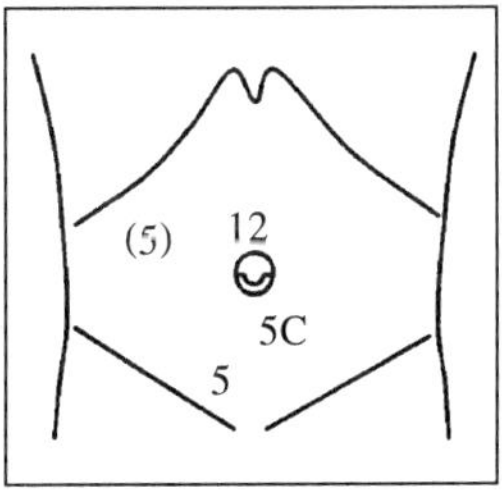

1. Make an umbilical incision and **enter** peritoneal cavity via open entry technique
2. Place trocar (e.g., 12 mm) and insufflate abdomen to create **pneumoperitoneum**
3. Example of port arrangement: Place two 5 mm **suprapubic** trocars (one for 5 mm laparoscope and one for dissector/grasper), optional one in right mid-upper abdomen (parentheses)
4. Examine peritoneal cavity and **assess** whether appendix is inflamed, purulent, gangrenous, perforated
5. **Mobilize** appendix
6. Take down **mesoappendix** with clips or endoscopic stapler
7. **Staple/divide** base of appendix; or **ligate** appendix with two endo-loops, then place 3rd endo-loop distally, **divide** appendix between proximal 2 and distal endo-loops
8. **Remove** appendix through umbilical port site using specimen bag or within trocar so as to avoid contaminating trocar site
9. Note: If appendix is *not* grossly inflamed, must **R/O** Crohn's, diverticulitis, Meckel's diverticulitis, GYN path. in women, perf'd. gastric or duodenal ulcer, cholecystitis
10. **Irrigate** copiously, close incisions, and place drain if RLQ abscess present; close fascia of all trocar sites larger than 5 mm

Risks: Hemorrhage, bowel injury (mechanical/thermal), CO_2 embolism, abscess, wound infection, postop ileus, trocar site hernia

Biliary Bypass [8]

Indications:

Urgent: Cholangitis not amenable to percutaneous or endoscopic drainage
Elective: Biliary obstruction due to neoplasm, stricture

Setup: Position = supine; Foley; NGT

Procedure:

1. Perform right subcostal or upper-midline abd incision; **explore** abdomen
2. Perform **cholecystectomy** (if GB present)
3. Identify and **expose** the dilated common hepatic duct (for hepaticojejunostomy) or common bile duct (choledochojejunostomy) distal to the obstruction
4. Perform **Kocher maneuver** to mobilize duodenum **OR** mobilize **Roux-en-Y** jejunal limb (if duodenal obstruction)
5. If performing side-to-side anastomosis, **anchor** bowel to bile duct with row of interrupted sutures
6. For side-to-side anastomosis, make ~ 2 cm longitudinal **incision** in duct adjacent to suture line; gently dilate until free flow of bile achieved
7. Make ~ 2 cm longitudinal **incision** in bowel (adjacent to suture line)
8. Using absorbable suture, perform single-layer **anastomosis** of entire bowel wall to bile duct; alternatively, transect CBD, and suture end-to-side to duodenum or jejunum
9. Place **drain** near anastomosis
10. Irrigate and **CLOSE**

Postop: NG suction to avoid gastric distension

Risks: Hemorrhage, anastomotic leak, cholangitis, stricture, wound infection/dehiscence

Breast Biopsy, Excisional — Palpable Mass

Indications:

1. Newly recognized, non-cystic, palpable breast mass, ± associated suspicious mammographic finding, ± personal risk factors and/or family history of breast cancer, ± worrisome findings on physical examination
2. Indeterminate, suspicious, or negative reports on fine needle biopsy
3. Failure of cystic mass to completely resolve after aspiration
4. Failure of suspected breast infection to resolve despite appropriate antibiotic therapy
5. Clinically and radiographically benign lesion in a patient with risk factors

Setup: Position = supine with arm extended on an arm board

Procedure:

1. Make curvilinear **incision** along Langer's lines, in a location and direction such that the scar could be included in any further surgery
2. **Palpate** lesion through wound
3. **Dissect** away from surrounding tissues and remove
4. **Orient** excised nodule and mark appropriately with sutures (e.g., long = lateral, short = superior)
5. Establish **hemostasis**
6. **Close** breast defect with interrupted sutures (optional)
7. Close **skin** with deep dermal and subcuticular sutures

Risks: Hemorrhage, hematoma/seroma, infection

Breast Biopsy, Excisional — Needle-Localization

Indications: Nonpalpable mammographic abnormality with suspicious characteristics

Setup: Position = supine with arm extended on board

Procedure:

1. Localizing **wire** is introduced into area of mammographic abnormality in radiology
2. View mammogram in **2 views** to discern location of mass with respect to the wire
3. Curvilinear **incision** in lines of skin cleavage (Langer's line) in area overlying lesion
4. Palpate wire and **remove** external portion out through wound
5. Circumferentially dissect out and **remove** suspected lesion using wire as guide
6. **Orient** excised nodule and mark with sutures
7. **X-ray** excised specimen to ensure complete removal of mammographic abnormality
8. Establish **hemostasis**
9. **Close** breast defect with interrupted sutures (optional)
10. Close **skin** with deep dermal and subcuticular sutures

Risks: Hemorrhage, hematoma/seroma, infection

Breast: Lumpectomy and Axillary Dissection

Indications: Biopsy-proven breast carcinoma

Setup: Position = supine with arm abducted at 90° angle on armboard; after draping, ipsilateral hemithorax, shoulder, and axilla should be readily accessible; anesthesia *without* paralysis preferred to aid identification/preservation of nerves

Procedure:

1. Make curvilinear **incision** along Langer's lines in a location and direction such that the scar could be included in any further surgery
2. Palpate lesion through wound, dissect away from surrounding tissues and **remove**
3. **Orient** excised nodule and mark appropriately with sutures (e.g., long = lateral, short = superior)
4. Make incision in inferior axilla between pectoralis and latissimus muscles, dissect down to **fat pad**, raise circumferential skin flaps
5. **Clipping and ligating** lymphatics/vessels, continue dissection anteriorly to pectoralis, posteriorly to latissimus dorsi, superiorly to axillary vein
6. **Early** in dissection, **identify and preserve**: **long thoracic** nerve by spreading posteriorly and sweeping against chest wall; **thoracodorsal** nerve, coursing through axilla toward latissiumus dorsi; **medial pectoral** nerve, representing the anteromedial extent of dissection along pectoralis muscle; **brachiocutaneous** nerve
7. Include all **nodal tissue** bordered by axillary vein superiorly, chest wall anteromedially, and latissimus dorsi posteriorly in specimen using sharp and blunt dissection; clip or ligate large vessels and lymphatics
8. Place **closed suction drain** within the axilla, bring out inferiorly
9. **Close** wounds in layers: interrupted sutures to obliterate breast defect; dermis with interrupted absorbable sutures; the skin with a subcuticular suture
10. Place drain to **bulb suction**

Postop: Drain remains in place for approximately one week; patient is to record drain output at home at regular intervals; may remove drains when the output is less than 20–30 ml per 24-hour period; antibiotics while drain is in place

Risks: Hemorrhage, hematoma/seroma, infection, ipsilateral upper extremity lymphedema, hypesthesias/paresthesias, winged scapula/shoulder apraxia

Breast: Modified Radical Mastectomy [8]

Indications: Biopsy-proven breast carcinoma

Setup: Position = supine with arm abducted at 90° angle on armboard; after draping, ipsilateral hemithorax, shoulder, and axilla should be readily accessible

Procedure:

1. Horizontal elliptical **incision** encompassing nipple-areolar complex and prior bx scar, extending from sternal margin medially to anterior margin lat. dorsi muscle laterally
2. Elevate superior & inferior **skin flaps**, encompassing all breast tissue within specimen while avoiding injury to overlying skin; during the dissection, skin flaps are retracted vertically by assistant using skin hooks
3. **Elevate** breast away from pectoralis major in medial to lateral fashion using electrocautery (include fascia on specimen side)
4. Clip or **ligate** perforating vessels; preserve pect. minor; carry dissection to anterior margin of latissimus dorsi muscle laterally
5. Include all **nodal tissue** bordered by axillary vein superiorly, chest wall anteromedially, and latissimus dorsi posteriorly in specimen using sharp and blunt dissection; clip or ligate large vessels and lymphatics
6. **Identify** and preserve long thoracic and thoracodorsal nerves: the long thoracic nerve runs in close proximity to the chest wall anterior to the subscapularis muscle; the thoracodorsal nerve lies lateral to the long thoracic nerve and medial to the thoracodorsal vessels, coursing inferolaterally towards the latissimus dorsi muscle
7. Place two **closed suction drains**, one overlying the pectoralis major muscle and the other within the axilla; bring out laterally through the inferior skin flap
8. **Close** wound in two layers: dermis with interrupted absorbable sutures; the skin with a subcuticular suture or staples
9. Place drains to **bulb suction**

Postop: Drains remain in place for approximately one week; patient is to record drain output at home at regular intervals; may remove drains when the output is less than 20–30 ml per 24-hour period; antibiotics while drain is in place

Risks: Ipsilateral upper extremity lymphedema, hypesthesias/paresthesias, winged scapula/shoulder apraxia and skin necrosis

Central Venous Catheter Placement, Subclavian — Tunneled Catheter or Port [9]

Indications: Long-term central venous access for parenteral nutrition, chemotherapy, chronic need for IV medications and/or phlebotomy, pheresis

Setup: Position = supine with roll beneath the thoracic spine, flat or slight Trendelenberg, with arms at sides, preferably pulled down toward feet; administer perioperative antibiotics; prep and drape to include bilateral infraclavicular and neck areas

Procedure:

1. **Insert needle** with bevel anterior in deltopectoral groove, 2 cm inferolateral to target area at point where clavicular head of the sternocleidomastoid inserts onto the clavicle
2. **Advance** needle under clavicle toward target area keeping syringe parallel to the floor with intermittent aspiration until blood return; if no blood return, retract needle slowly with intermittent aspiration
3. Upon free return of blood, rotate 90° to place the bevel toward the heart and insert **guidewire** through the needle and advance to junction of SVC and RA under fluoroscopic guidance
4. Make stab incision adjacent to wire and counter-incision on anterior chest wall at planned catheter exit site or the port location, and **tunnel** intravascular end of catheter cephalad subcutaneously from the catheter exit site to guidewire exit site
5. In the case of subcutaneous **port** placement, a subcutaneous **pocket** is created bluntly and the port is secured to the pectoral fascia with 3–4 circumferential interrupted non-absorbable sutures
6. Measure catheter, cut to the appropriate length, and **position** so that the fibrous cuff is located ~ 2 cm from the exit site in the subcutaneous tract (note: placing further from catheter exit site allows more room for re-positioning catheter if needed, but makes eventual removal of the catheter more difficult)
7. Place dilator/sheath assembly over wire, dilate tract to vein, remove dilator and insert the **catheter** through sheath, peel away sheath, and confirm position with fluoroscopy
8. **Close** infraclavicular wound with a single absorbable subcutaneous stitch, close port incision (if present) in two layers, secure catheter with 1–2 nonabsorbable sutures at exit, dress wounds/exit site
9. Aspirate and **flush** all catheter ports with heparin-containing solutions
10. Obtain postoperative **chest film** to document catheter position and identify complications (always check yourself)

Risks: Hemorrhage (incl. perforation of SVC with dilator, cardiac rupture), pneumothorax, improper position, nerve injury, chylothorax, arrhythmia, infection (site, port/tract, line sepsis), DVT/PE/septic thrombophlebitis

Cholecystectomy — Open [8]

Indications:

1. Symptomatic cholelithiasis: biliary colic, acute cholecystitis ± evidence of choledocholithiasis, or h/o cholangitis
2. Acute acalculous cholecystitis
3. Second-line treatment for the above indications in patients: in whom initial laparoscopic attempt failed, prompting conversion; or with extensive h/o abdominal surgery, especially involving the upper abdomen or RUQ
4. Gallbladder cancer

Setup: Position = supine; NGT for gastric decompression

Procedure:

1. Right subcostal or upper midline **incision**
2. Take down subhepatic adhesions, retract liver and **expose** gallbladder, place self-retaining retractor (e.g., Buchwalter)
3. **Incise** peritoneum at inferior aspect of gallbladder (may dissect GB from GB fossa at this point if anterograde approach is preferred)
4. Grasp gallbladder infundibulum with clamp, and retract laterally and cephalad to **open triangle** of Calot (decompression of gallbladder by needle aspiration may be helpful prior to this step)
5. Identify cystic duct, doubly clamp, with distal clamp adequately proximal to CBD confluence; divide **cystic duct** between clamps using transfixing suture for distal stump (if indicated, may perform cholangiogram prior to ligating duct, for instance, if there is a history of gallstone pancreatitis or jaundice or elevated alk phos/bilirubin, or to clarify anatomy)
6. If performing **cholangiogram**, thread catheter into cystic duct and clip gently to hold in place, connect to three-way stopcock with a syringe of saline and another of contrast, clear all bubbles and flush with saline, place pt flat or in mild Trendelenberg position, infuse contrast while obtaining plain film or fluoroscopy
7. Identify, doubly clamp, divide, and ligate **cystic artery**
8. Carefully dissect **gallbladder** away from its hepatic bed using electrocautery (if not performed in step 3)
9. Ensure **hemostasis**, consider closed-suction drain in gallbladder bed in cases of marginal/poor hemostasis or soilage with grossly purulent material
10. **Close** fascia in two layers with absorbable suture, reapproximate skin edges with staples or subcuticular suture

Risks: Biliary ductal injury (right hepatic duct, common duct; inadvertent tearing, resection, division, clipping, injury resulting in stricture), bile leakage, hemorrhage, spilled stones, subhepatic/intraperitoneal abscess, injury to adjacent organs

Cholecystectomy — Laparoscopic [10]

Indications:

1. Symptomatic cholelithiasis: biliary colic, acute cholecystitis ± evidence of choledocholithiasis, h/o gallstone pancreatitis, h/o cholangitis
2. Acute acalculous cholecystitis
3. Patients with h/o sickle cell disease and frequent abdominal crises

Setup: Position = supine; NGT; SCD boots

Procedure:

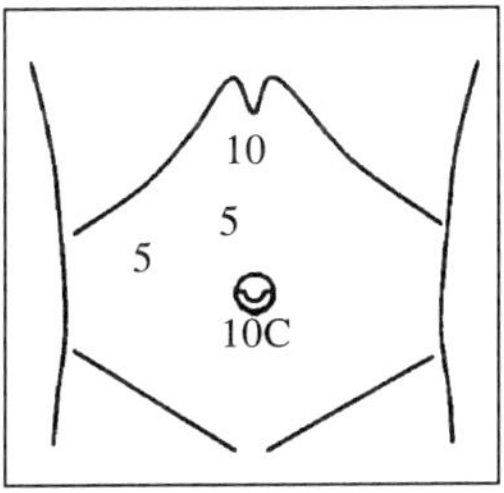

1. Vertical or transverse supra- or infraumbilical 1–2 cm **incision**, incise fascia (vertically) and place #1 vicryl traction sutures through each side of fascia
2. Enter fascia/peritoneum under direct visualization with Hasson trocar and insufflate with CO_2 to 15 mm Hg (open technique) to create **pneumoperitoneum**
3. Introduce **laparoscope**, explore abdominal cavity; place pt in reverse Trendelenberg position and airplane to the left
4. Place one 10 mm upper midline and two 5 mm right subcostal operative **trocars** under laparoscopic visualization
5. Gallbladder **retraction**: fundus in cephalad direction over liver, infundibulum laterally and inferiorly, thus opening up triangle of Calot
6. Isolate **cystic duct** in close proximity to infundibulum, clip twice on pt side/once on gallbladder side, and divide (may perform cholangiogram using cholangiocath prior to division of cystic duct, as indicated [see open cholecystectomy])
7. Isolate **cystic artery**, clip twice on pt side and once on gallbladder side, and divide
8. Dissect **gallbladder** away from intrahepatic fossa, remove through one of 10 mm ports (may place within specimen retrieval bag prior to removal)
9. Irrigate operative site with saline, ensure **hemostasis**, consider closed suction drain placement (see open cholecystectomy for indications)
10. **Close** fascia at umbilical site with heavy figure-of-eight absorbable suture and/or tie traction stitches together; close skin with subcuticular sutures, wound tapes

Postop: No routine labs postop unless concerned about intraop complication, CBD stone(s), or signif pain

Risks: Biliary ductal injury (right hepatic duct, common duct; inadvertent tearing, resection, division, clipping, injury resulting in stricture), bile leakage biloma, hemorrhage, spilled stones, subhepatic/intraperitoneal abscess, injury to adjacent organs (during port placement or via electrocautery injury). Note: performance of intraoperative cholangiography does not decrease the incidence of biliary ductal injury.

Colostomy/Ileostomy [4,8]

Indications:

Urgent — Decompression of large bowel or distal small bowel obstruction; protection of distal suture lines in unprepped cases
Elective — Protection of high-risk, distal reconstructions; severe and refractory incontinence, constipation, perirectal disease, or sacral decubiti

Setup: Mark abdominal wall for stoma/bag location preop when possible (should pass through rectus muscle, be in easily managed location); Position = supine; Foley; NGT

Procedure:

1. **Laparotomy** or **laparoscopy** to expose desired segment of bowel
2. **Excise** small, round piece of skin in the vicinity of stoma
3. Expose fascia and make a cruciate or longitudinal **incision**, large enough to be just snug around bowel (e.g., two fingers in case of colostomy)
4. **Mark** proximal/distal limbs if ileostomy (e.g., dark suture = distal)
5. Carefully **deliver** colon/ileum into wound (additional, separate incision may be necessary for mobilization)

Loop

5. Pass **red rubber catheter** (or stiff rod) through mesenteric defect (this is removed several days postop)
6. **Suture serosa** of bowel to fascia with interrupted sutures (optional)
7. To **mature** in operating room, open loop of bowel with linear incision (in case of ileostomy, make transverse incision on *distal* side of loop)
8. **Suture circumferentially** full-thickness bowel edge to dermis with interrupted absorbable sutures, and for ileostomy evert over proximal limb to create raised nipple
9. Apply **ostomy bag**

End

5. **Divide** bowel with linear stapling device, leaving at least 4 cm of proximal bowel outside the skin; return distal loop to abdomen
6. **Suture serosa** of proximal loop to fascia with interrupted sutures (optional)
7. Excise staple line and **mature** to skin with absorbable sutures (for *Brooke* ileostomy, sutures include bite of serosa 1–2 cm proximal to end, full-thickness bite of intestinal wall at edge, and dermis)
8. Apply **ostomy bag**

Postop: Ostomy RN for teaching, supplies; careful fluid management post-ileostomy

Risks: Hemorrhage, SBO, stoma ischemia/necrosis/dehiscence, prolapse, parastomal hernia

Colorectal: Right Hemicolectomy †

Indications:

Urgent — Right colon hemorrhage, ischemia, or obstructing lesion/process (benign or malignant)
Elective — Benign or malignant neoplasm or stricture

Setup: Position = supine; Foley; NGT; SCD boots

Procedure:

1. **Midline** abd incision, **explore** abdomen (esp. liver and peritoneal surfaces, if malignancy)
2. **Mobilize** ascending colon by incising white line of Toldt, take down lateral attachments through avascular plane using gentle counter-traction to mobilize mesentery
3. **Score** mesentery with cautery at margins of resection
4. Make a window at mesenteric border of ileum just proximal to ileocecal junction, and **divide ileum** (proximal margin of resection) with linear cutting stapler
5. **Divide mesentery** between clamps along previously scored lines, with particular attention to ileocolic and right colic vascular pedicles
6. Make a window at mesenteric border of colon near hepatic flexure (distal margin of resection), and **divide colon** with linear cutting stapler
7. Using stapler, **anastomose** terminal ileum and transverse colon (e.g., functional end-to-end, i.e., with lumens oriented toward same direction)
8. Inspect neo-lumen for bleeding and use stapler to **complete** anastomosis
9. **Close mesenteric defect**, taking caution not to close resulting defect and thus compromise blood supply
10. **Close** abdomen

Risks: Hemorrhage, MI, pneumonia, SBO, wound infection/dehiscence, anastomotic leak

† Similar steps are used for other segmental colectomies

Colorectal: Low Anterior Resection

Indications:

Urgent — Rectosigmoid hemorrhage, abscess, ischemia, or stricture
Elective — Benign or malignant neoplasm or stricture

Setup: Position = modified lithotomy; Foley; NGT; SCD boots

Procedure:

1. Midline abd incision; **explore** abdomen (esp. liver and peritoneum, if malignancy)
2. **Mobilize** left colon (by taking down lateral attachments), and splenic flexure, and take omentum down from distal transverse colon
3. **Ligate** the IMA at its origin (provided adequate collateral circulation via marginal artery is anticipated), left colic off IMA, and IMV just below pancreas
4. Create window along mesenteric border of proximal line of resection, and apply linear cutting stapler to **divide colon** at this point, pack bowels into upper abdomen (consider placing self-retaining retractor), and turn attention to pelvic dissection
5. **Score** mesentery along planned margins of resection, continuing dissection of colon/rectum down toward pelvic floor, ligating/dividing vascular pedicles
6. Identify and **avoid** ureters and presacral venous plexus
7. In males, **anteriorly** divide Denonvillier's fascia posterior to the prostate; in females, divide the cul-de-sac and separate the rectum from the urinary bladder and vagina
8. Divide **distal** rectum at least 2 cm below tumor using stapler
9. **Reanastomose** bowel with EEA stapler (ensure two intact rings of bowel); perform proctoscopy, fill pelvis with saline, insufflate air and confirm integrity of anastomosis
10. Irrigate, consider placing closed suction drain, and **close** abdomen

Risks: Hemorrhage, MI, pneumonia, SBO, wound infection/dehiscence, anastomotic leak, sexual dysfunction

Colorectal: Abdominoperineal Resection [4,8]

Indications:

Urgent — Rectal hemorrhage, abscess, ischemia, or stricture
Elective — Benign or malignant neoplasm or stricture

Setup: Mark pt for colostomy preop; Position = lithotomy; Foley; NGT; SCD boots

Procedure:

1. Midline abd incision; **explore** abdomen (esp. liver and peritoneum, if malignancy)
2. **Mobilize** left colon (by taking down lateral attachments)
3. **Ligate** the IMA at its origin (provided adequate collateral circulation via marginal artery), left colic off IMA, and IMV just below pancreas
4. Create window along mesenteric border of proximal line of resection, and apply linear cutting stapler to **divide colon** at this point, pack bowels into upper abdomen (consider placing self-retaining retractor)
5. **Score** mesentery along planned margins of resection, identify and **avoid** ureters and presacral venous plexus
6. Dissect **laterally** to the pelvic sidewalls and carry dissection down to pelvic floor, carefully identifying and avoiding ureters
7. In **perineum**, make elliptical incision around anus into ischioanal fossae, dissect circumferentially coming through levator ani laterally, flush with the pelvic sidewalls
8. Bring **specimen** out through perineal incision; irrigate copiously and close perineal wound in layers with *absorbable* suture
9. Perform end **colostomy**
10. Irrigate, consider placing closed suction drain, and **close** abdomen

Risks: Hemorrhage, MI, pneumonia, SBO, wound infection/dehiscence, pelvic abscess, sexual dysfunction

Colorectal: Proctocolectomy with Ileal Pouch-Anal Anastomosis [4,8]

Indications:

Familial polyposis syndromes, ulcerative colitis

Setup: Mark pt preoperatively for ileostomy; Position = lithotomy; Foley; NGT; SCD boots

Procedure:

1. Expose anal canal with **Hill-Ferguson** retractors and identify dentate line
2. Perform circumferential **mucosal incision** just above dentate line and develop plane between rectal mucosa and internal sphincter muscle upward for ~ 2 cm
3. Use 3-0 chromic suture to **oversew** distal mucosal edge
4. Midline abdominal incision; **explore** abdomen
5. Identify ileocecal valve and perform total abdominal **colectomy** (from just proximal to ileocecal valve to anus)
6. Remove specimen from peritoneal cavity and carefully **mobilize** terminal ileum
7. Fashion **J-pouch** from terminal ileum by making 15–20 cm loop with stapler
8. **Anastomose** apex of pouch to dentate line with interrupted 3-0 absorbable sutures
9. Perform diverting loop **ileostomy** to protect anastomosis
10. Irrigate, consider placing closed suction drain, and **close** abdomen

Risks: Hemorrhage, splenic injury requiring splenectomy, MI, pneumonia, SBO, wound infection/dehiscence, anastomotic leak, incontinence

Colorectal: Transanal Excision of Rectal Tumor

Indications:

Benign or malignant neoplasms ≤ 10 cm from anal verge

Setup: Position = prone jack-knife or lithotomy

Procedure:

1. Spread buttocks with **tape** and prep perianal area and buttocks widely
2. **Expose** anus/rectum with Hill-Ferguson retractor (or circumferentially placed traction stitches, etc.), and identify dentate line
3. **Grasp** mucosa distal to lesion with Allis clamp
4. While lifting with Allis, **excise** full thickness of rectum with electrocautery or Metzenbaum scissors (certain/high lesion may require operating proctoscope ± snare); obtain at least 1 cm margin of normal tissue if feasible
5. **Orient** specimen for pathologist by pinning to a cork board
6. **Close** defect with running layer of absorbable suture
7. **Proctoscopy** may be performed to verify complete excision and hemostasis

Risks: Hemorrhage, pelvic abscess/sepsis, fecal incontinence

Common Bile Duct Exploration/Sphincterotomy

Indication: Elevation in liver function tests (or other evidence suggesting choledocholithiasis) in the setting of open cholecystectomy or during laparotomy for other reasons

Setup: Position = supine; foley, NGT

Procedure — CBD Exploration:

1. Upper midline or right subcostal **incision**
2. **Pack** bowels out of portal area
3. Place 4-0 silk **stay sutures** into CBD
4. The **gallbladder** may be removed at this point if it is large and/or obscuring view of the CBD or may be removed after CBD exploration
5. Make a 1 cm longitudinal **choledochotomy** between stay sutures
6. Explore CBD with **choledochoscope**
7. Pass **stone** scoop (8–15 mm) into the duct, first distally, then proximally into each hepatic duct. (stone may be cleared by flushing distally through ampulla, or retrieving with fogarty balloon catheter or by basket retrieval)
8. Place a **T-tube** (14–16 fr) into the opening and close CBD around tube with 4-0 absorbable sutures
9. Perform **cholangiogram**
10. Bring **T-tube** out a separate stab incision and **close** abdomen

Procedure — Sphincterotomy/Sphincteroplasty:

1. **Incision/Exposure** as above
2. **Kocher** maneuver to mobilize duodenum
3. Place stay sutures opposite to the site of ampulla and **open duodenum** longitudinally 2–3 cm
4. Visualize ampulla and make vertical incision (at ~ 11 o'clock) to open the ampulla (**sphincterotomy**), and suture the duodenum to bile duct horizontally with absorbable sutures (**sphincteroplasty**)
5. **Close duodenum** transversely, place closed suction **drains**
6. **Close** abdomen

Postop: Leave T-tube in place at least 10–14 days, perform T-tube cholangiogram prior to removal

Risks: Biliary ductal injury, bile leak, hemorrhage, cholangitis, duodenal injury, spilled stones

Esophagectomy — Transhiatal (Orringer) [11]

Indication:

Esophageal cancer, Barrett's esophagus with dysplasia

Setup: Position = supine; Foley; NGT; A-line; CVP line ± Swan

Procedure:

1. Perform **upper midline** incision; **explore** abdomen
2. **Mobilize** stomach, preserving entire length of gastroepiploic vessels and dividing short gastric vessels; divide phrenoesophageal ligament anteriorly
3. Encircle intra-abdominal esophagus with **Penrose** drain and divide inferior aspect of gastrohepatic ligament
4. Perform **pyloromyotomy** or **pyloroplasty**
5. Dissect **lower** esophagus under direct visualization, clipping feeding vessels
6. Perform left **cervical** incision along sternocleidomastoid; dissect posteriorly down to esophagus using blunt finger dissection and avoiding recurrent laryngeal nerve anteriorly
7. Pass sponge-stick through cervical incision and hand through hiatus to complete blunt dissection of **retroesophageal** space
8. Ligate and **divide** cervical esophagus; peel mid-thoracic esophagus from anterior structures; divide stomach (at least 4–6 cm distal margin) and remove specimen through abdomen
9. Mobilize stomach up to neck and **anastomose** cervical esophagus to proximal end of stomach using interrupted sutures (must be tension-free)
10. Place **J-tube** (see J-tube placement), cervical closed-suction **drain**, **chest tube**(s) if pleural space(s) entered; **close** both incisions

Postop: Gastric decompression; barium swallow study POD 4-5 to √ anastomosis prior to PO intake

Risks: Hemorrhage, anastomotic leak, recurrent laryngeal nerve injury, MI, pneumonia, SBO, reflux/aspiration, anastomotic stricture, wound infection/dehiscence

Esophagectomy — Thoraco-abdominal (Ivor-Lewis) [12]

Indications:

Urgent — Esophageal perforation
Elective — Mid- to lower-third esophageal cancer

Setup: Position = supine; Foley; NGT; A-line; CVP ± Swan

Procedure:

1. Perform **upper midline** incision; **explore** abdomen
2. **Mobilize** stomach, preserving entire length of gastroepiploic vessels and dividing short gastric vessels; divide phrenoesophageal ligament anteriorly
3. Encircle intra-abdominal esophagus with **Penrose** drain and divide inferior aspect of gastrohepatic ligament; perform **pyloromyotomy** or **pyloroplasty**
4. Dissect **lower** esophagus under direct visualization, clipping feeding vessels
5. **Divide** stomach and **deliver** into chest through hiatus; **close** abdomen
6. Reposition patient and perform right posterolateral **thoracotomy** through the 5th or 6th intercostal space
7. Mobilize esophagus around tumor and **transect** as far proximally as possible, and remove specimen
8. **Anastomose** esophagus to apex of stomach using EEA stapler
9. Place **chest tube**
10. **Close** thoracotomy incision

Postop: Gastric decompression; barium swallow study on POD 4-5 to √ anastomosis prior to PO intake

Risks: Hemorrhage, anastomotic leak/mediastinitis, MI, pneumonia, SBO, reflux/aspiration, anastomotic stricture, wound infection/dehiscence

Gastrectomy — Total [8]

Indications:

1. Gastric adenocarcinoma or sarcoma with no distant metastases (curative intent)
2. Advanced gastric cancer (palliative intent)
3. Intractable ulcer diathesis such as 2° to pancreatic neuroendocrine tumors (unresectable gastrinoma)
4. Gastric lymphoma

Setup: Position = supine

Procedure:

1. **Upper midline** abdominal incision, **explore** abdomen for metastases or local invasion
2. Mobilize stomach and proximal duodenum; ligate right gastroepiploic vessels on inferior margin of duodenum, and right gastric vessels on superior margin of duodenum, then **divide duodenum** distal to pylorus (stapled or handsewn closure)
3. **Mobilize** left lobe of liver by dividing left triangular ligament and gastrohepatic ligament
4. **Ligate** and divide left gastric vessels, gastrosplenic ligament (sparing spleen), and left gastroepiploic vessels
5. Isolate distal esophagus, anchor outer muscular layer of esophagus to crus; clamp and **divide esophagus** above G-E junction, and remove stomach
6. Mobilize and **divide jejunum** (with stapler or scalpel) approximately 30 cm beyond ligament of Treitz
7. Perform end-to-side **esophagojejunostomy** in two layers (absorbable suture for mucosa, non-absorbable suture for muscularis) or with stapler (EEA)
8. Mobilize distal jejunum to esophagus through an incision in the transverse mesocolon (retrocolic), complete the **Roux-en-Y** anastomosis by constructing an end-to-side jejuno-jejunostomy, close defects in the mesocolon
9. **Consider** placing nasojejunal tube (NJT), feeding J-tube, and closed suction drains
10. **Close** abdomen

Postop: Do not replace NJT if inadvertently removed
Barium swallow 5–7 days postop to R/O leak
Advance diet to post-gastrectomy diet (6 small meals/day); will require supplemental B_{12} 100–200 mcg IM q month.

Risks: Hemorrhage anastomotic leak or stricture; dumping syndrome, pernicious anemia duodenal stump blowout

Gastric: Vagotomy and Antrectomy [4,8,13,14]

Indications:

Peptic ulcer disease refractory to medical management and/or associated with complications including gastric outlet obstruction, bleeding, and perforation

Setup: Fluid resuscitation, NPO, bowel prep, administer perioperative antibiotics

Procedure:

1. **Upper midline** incision, **explore** abdomen
2. **Expose** the esophageal hiatus, mobilizing the left lobe of the liver if necessary
3. **Incise** the gastrohepatic ligament over the esophagus, encircle esophagus and locate anterior and posterior vagus trunks
4. **Vagotomy**: mobilize both vagal trunks and excise a 1 cm segment of each between clips and send to pathology for confirmation
5. Perform a complete **Kocher** maneuver
6. Further **mobilize** the stomach by dividing the gastrohepatic ligament, the splenocolic ligament, and detaching the greater omentum from the greater curvature, taking care to identify and protect the duodenal blood supply
7. If indicated, biopsy ulcer bed via high anterior gastrotomy; if benign diagnosis confirmed, identify line of stomach transection (incisura angularis to greater curvature), apply bowel clamps and **divide stomach** sharply or with stapler
8. Identify pylorus and **divide duodenum** distal to perforation or area of inflammation with a stapler
9. Perform **anastomosis** of duodenum (Billroth I) or loop of jejunum (Billroth II) to dependent portion of gastric remnant by hand sewing, with linear stapler, or with EEA stapler
10. Irrigate abdomen, consider NG tube placement and **close** abdomen in a routine fashion

Postop: NPO (± NG tube) for 3–5 days, advance diet with return of bowel. Following recovery, H. *pylori* treatment and endoscopic follow-up if indicated

Risks: Hemorrhage, ulcer re-bleeding, gastroparesis, bowel obstruction, duodenal stump blowout (with Billroth II), fistula, leak, infection, recurrent peptic ulceration, dumping syndrome, post-vagotomy diarrhea, malabsorption, bile reflux gastritis

Gastric: Truncal Vagotomy and Pyloroplasty (Heineke-Mikulicz) [4,8,14]

Indications:

1. Peptic ulcer disease refractory to medical management
2. In combination with repair of a perforated ulcer in a patient previously treated medically for peptic ulcer disease

Setup: Fluid resuscitation, NPO, bowel prep

Procedure:

1. **Upper midline** incision, **explore** abdomen
2. **Expose** the esophageal hiatus, mobilizing the left lobe of the liver if necessary
3. **Incise** the gastrohepatic ligament over the esophagus
4. **Encircle** esophagus with Penrose, retract anteriorly, identify anterior and posterior vagal trunks
5. **Vagotomy**: mobilize both vagal trunks and excise a 1 cm segment of each between clips and send to pathology for confirmation
6. Identify the pylorus and perform **Kocher** maneuver on proximal duodenum
7. Place **stay sutures** on the medial and lateral walls of the pylorus at the midpoint of the planned longitudinal pyloric incision
8. **Incise** the **pylorus** longitudinally
9. **Close** defect **transversely** in single layer with single layer of vicryl or silk suture, using the stay sutures to orient the tissue edges
10. Irrigate abdomen, consider NGT placement, and **close**

Postop: NPO (± NG tube) until return of bowel function; following recovery, H. pylori treatment and endoscopic follow-up if indicated

Risks: Hemorrhage/ulcer re-bleeding, gastroparesis, bowel obstruction, fistula, leak, infection, recurrent peptic ulceration, dumping syndrome, post-vagotomy diarrhea, malabsorption, bile reflux gastritis

Gastroduodenostomy — Billroth I [4,8]

Indications:

Urgent — Gastric outlet obstruction
Elective — Reconstruction following gastric resection for benign disease (most physiologic reconstruction); conversion from BII for dumping syndrome

Setup: Position = supine; Foley; NGT

Procedure:

1. **Upper-midline** abd incision; **explore** abdomen
2. **Mobilize** stomach by ligating and dividing the gastrocolic ligament and gastric vessels distal to point of planned transection
3. Perform **vagotomy** (if indicated)
4. **Kocher maneuver** to mobilize duodenum (BI contraindicated in presence of marked inflammation)
5. **Divide** the duodenum (distal to the obstruction, if present)
6. **Check** that the NGT is pulled back and **divide** the stomach (along line from lesser to greater curvature) between non-crushing clamps or with linear cutting stapler, remove specimen
7. **Partially close** the gastric pouch at the lesser curvature with linear stapler and/or sutures
8. Perform stapled or single-layer hand-sewn **anastomosis** of stomach to duodenum
9. **Confirm** patency, hemostasis, absence of tension (and position of NGT if placed)
10. **Close**: Irrigate; consider retention sutures in setting of severe malnutrition or medical condition associated with poor wound healing

Postop: NPO (± NG tube) until return of bowel function

Risks: Hemorrhage, anastomotic leak, wound infection/dehiscence, bile reflux, delayed gastric emptying

Gastrojejunostomy — Billroth II [4,8]

Indications:

Urgent — Gastric outlet obstruction
Elective — Reconstruction following gastric resection for malignancy or peptic ulcer disease

Setup: Position = supine; Foley; NGT

Procedure:

1. **Upper-midline** abd incision; **explore** abdomen
2. **Mobilize** stomach and first portion of duodenum by ligating and dividing the gastrocolic ligament and gastric vessels distal to point of planned transection
3. Perform **vagotomy** (if indicated)
4. **Divide** the duodenum just distal to the pylorus; close duodenal stump using linear stapling device and/or suture, consider placement of duodenostomy tube if duodenum is very inflamed or fibrotic
5. **Divide** the stomach between non-crushing clamps or with linear cutting stapler, remove specimen
6. **Close** the gastric pouch with linear stapler and/or sutures
7. Manipulate stomach down through a window in the transverse mesocolon (retrocolic) adjacent to **loop** of proximal **jejunum**
8. Perform stapled or 2 layer, hand-sewn **anastomosis** of the jejunum to the posterior gastric wall
9. **Confirm** patency, adequate blood supply, absence of tension, and hemostasis
10. **Close**: Irrigate; consider retention sutures in setting of severe malnutrition or condition associated with poor wound healing

Postop: NPO (± NG tube) until return of bowel function

Risks: Hemorrhage, anastomotic leak, wound infection/dehiscence, dumping syndrome, duodenal stump blowout

Gastrojejunostomy — Roux-en-Y [8]

Indications:

Urgent: Gastric outlet obstruction
Elective: Reconstruction following gastric resection for malignancy or peptic ulcer disease; revision of BI or BII for bile reflux
Caution: Contraindicated in setting of gastroparesis

Setup: Position = supine; Foley; NGT; ± CVP, A-line

Procedure:

1. Perform **gastric resection**, if necessary, as described for BII gastrojej. (Steps 1–6)
2. **Divide** the jejunum with a stapler ~ 40 cm distal to LOT
3. Manipulate stomach down through a window in the transverse mesocolon (retrocolic) and position adjacent to distal limb of divided **jejunum**
4. Perform a side-to-side stapled or hand-sewn **anastomosis** of the jejunal limb to the posterior gastric wall
5. Perform an end-to-side **anastomosis** of the proximal limb of the divided jejunum to a loop of jejunum ~ 40 cm distal to the gastrojejunostomy
6. **Confirm** patency, hemostasis, and absence of tension
7. **Close**: Irrigate; consider retention sutures in setting of severe malnutrition or medical condition associated with poor wound healing

Postop: NPO until return of bowel function

Risks: Hemorrhage, anastomotic leak, wound infection/dehiscence, dumping syndrome

Gastrostomy — Open (Stamm) [4]

Indications:

Long-term feeding access; long-term gastric decompression; to anchor stomach following paraesophageal/hiatal hernia repair

Setup: Supine

Procedure:

1. Short **upper midline** incision approximately 6–8 cm (Alternatively, may use LUQ incision, 4–5 cm incision transecting the rectus 2 fingerbreadths below the costal margin)
2. Retract stomach inferiorly with Babcock clamps; choose site midway between lesser and greater curvatures on anterior stomach and place 2-0 silk **pursestring** suture
3. Place an additional **concentric** 2-0 silk pursestring suture around the first
4. Make stab wound in LUQ abdominal wall, and carefully pass 18-22 Fr **gastric tube** (or Malecott catheter) into abdomen
5. Make stab incision in stomach with cautery, **insert** catheter into stomach and inflate balloon with saline
6. **Tie** inner pursestring to invaginate gastric serosa around tube; tie outer pursestring
7. **Tack** gastric wall to inside of anterior abdominal wall with four interrupted 2-0 silk sutures
8. **Close** midline incision in standard fashion (close peritoneum/fascia with interrupted or running 0 non-absorbable suture)
9. **Secure** G-tube to skin of abdominal wall with 2-0 nonabsorbable suture

Postop: Place gastric tube to straight drainage (or cap) for 24–48 hours prior to starting feeds

Risks: Hemorrhage, injury to colon or other organ, tube displacement ± intra-abdominal soilage/peritonitis, abdominal wall erosion ± necrotizing fasciitis, minor site infection/cellulitis, erosion through the stomach wall

Gastrostomy — Percutaneous endoscopic gastronomy (PEG) [15]

Indications:

Long-term feeding access or need for long-term gastric decompression; may be preferred in patients who cannot tolerate general anesthesia

Setup: Supine; mouthguard for endoscope; prep and drape abdomen in standard fashion

Procedure:

1. Endoscopist — Place pediatric **gastroscope** through oropharynx, down esophagus and into stomach, examining mucosa along the way for strictures, ulcers, etc.
2. Endoscopist — **Insufflate** stomach with air and direct scope anteriorly
3. Darken room lights; Surgeon — Select spot on anterior abdominal wall in LUQ approximately 4–5 cm below costal margin, look for transmitted glow of endoscope on abd. wall indent with index finger; Endoscopist — confirm **clear indentation** of gastric wall
4. Surgeon — Infiltrate lidocaine at selected spot on abdominal wall and pass 16-gauge trocar/**needle** through abdominal wall and into stomach (briskly, but cautiously, and to depth appropriate for pt's body habitus), start passing braided wire through needle
5. Endoscopist — Pass **snare** through endoscope, lasso needle, pass braided wire through needle, and grasp wire with snare
6. Endoscopist — **Retrieve** endoscope and wire retrogradely out through mouth, attach G-tube to wire, lubricate with antibiotic ointment
7. Surgeon — **pull tube**/wire anterogradely through pharynx and esophagus into stomach, out through abdominal wall until appropriate markings on G-tube are visible externally (generally at ~ 2–4 cm marking)
8. Surgeon — Place **retainer disk** over G-tube and snug down against abdominal wall with betadine gauze between disk and skin
9. Surgeon — Using Kelly clamp, thread **sleeve** (if kit requires) over tube to secure disk in place
10. Surgeon — **Trim tube** to appropriate length and cap

Postop: Place to straight drain for 24 hours; then begin small bolus feeding. Advance to full support as tolerated. Loosen disc at 4–5 days to avoid gastric wall erosion (longer if on steroids, malnourished, or has poor wound healing) - controversial

Risks: Hemorrhage, injury to colon or other organ, tube displacement ± intra-abdominal soilage/peritonitis, abdominal wall erosion ± necrotizing fasciitis, minor site infection/cellulitis

Hepatic Resection [4,16]

Indications:

1. Hepatic adenoma — increased risk of rupture and hemorrhage, possible occult malignancy; 2. Hepatocellular carcinoma — Childs class A; 3. Selected metastatic cancer deposits; 4. Symptomatic hemangiomas or simple cysts; 5. Resectable cholangiocarcinoma (no involvement of porta hepatis); 6. Selected primary hepatic malignancies

Setup: Position = supine and slight reverse Trendelenberg; prep from nipples to pubis

Procedure:

1. Right subcostal **incision** extending across midline into left subcostal region (hockey-stick); optional midline extension cranially to xyphoid
2. **Explore** abdomen for evidence of extrahepatic disease or lesions missed by preop evaluation; perform intraoperative ultrasound; abort procedure if extra-hepatic disease or unresectable lesions are found
3. **Cholecystectomy**, then **mobilize** liver by taking down triangular and falciform ligaments
4. Obtain control of portal triad and hepatic vein with vessel loops/Rumel tourniquets; ligate and **divide** hepatic duct(s) first, followed by hepatic artery(ies) (beware of aberrant anatomy)
5. Ligate and **divide** segmental portal vein(s) between two Cooley clamps
6. **Clamp** hepatic vein; demarcation between right and left guides initial dissection
7. **Dissect** through hepatic parenchyma with Kelly clamp, CUSA, cautery, and/or laser; larger vessels and ducts should be ligated or clipped, and hepatic vein is taken from within the liver parenchyma (may ligate or use vascular load of linear cutting stapler); need 2 cm margin around tumor
8. **Examine** remaining lobe for bile leak or bleeding, using argon coagulation or suture ligation to achieve hemostasis; mobilize omentum to cover raw surface of liver
9. Place closed-suction **drains** in the right upper quadrant
10. **Close** fascia with a durable non-absorbable suture; close subcutaneous tissue and skin

Risks: Hemorrhage, bile leak, hepatic insufficiency, abscess

Hernia Repair, Inguinal — Bassini [8]

Indications:

Elective — Symptomatic inguinal hernia
Urgent — Incarcerated or strangulated inguinal hernia

Setup: Position = supine

Procedure:

1. If **local**/MAC anesthesia, administer 1% lidocaine to line of skin incision and base of ilioinguinal nerve near anterior superior iliac spine; test sensation
2. Oblique **incision** extending from medial to the anterior superior iliac spine to pubis; incise Scarpa's fascia and expose external oblique fascia
3. Infiltrate 1% lidocaine beneath external oblique fascia (if local anesthesia); incise **external oblique** fascia in the direction of its fibers and extend *through* external ring; identify and protect ilioinguinal nerve
4. Bluntly separate **spermatic cord** from surrounding structures and encircle it with a Penrose drain
5. Divide cremasteric fibers with sharp and blunt dissection, **free** hernia sac (anteromedial to cord for indirect) up to internal ring; open sac if indirect, and for either type reduce sac contents into abdomen (*beware* of sliding hernias)
6. For indirect hernia, ligate sac at its neck, and excise excess; for either type, **reduce** sac and secure in reduced position with Z-stitch
7. **Reinforce** internal ring and inguinal floor by approximating iliopubic tract (medial to inguinal ligament) to transversus abdominis aponeurosis above and below internal ring using 2-0 polypropylene (or other nonabsorbable suture) — *beware* of femoral vessels
8. **Suture** conjoined tendon to medial edge of inguinal ligament without excessive tension using 2-0 polypropylene (relaxing incisions in rectus sheath may be necessary)
9. **Reapproximate** edges of the external oblique fascia
10. **Close** Scarpa's fascia, then skin with subcuticular suture or staples; retract testis into scrotal sac

Risks/Results: Inguinal nerve injury, neuroma or neuritis, scrotal hematoma, testicular ischemia/loss, hernia recurrence

Hernia Repair, Inguinal — Lichtenstein [8]

Indications:

Elective — Symptomatic inguinal hernia
Urgent — Incarcerated inguinal hernia

Setup: Position = supine

Procedure:

1. If **local**/MAC anesthesia, administer 1% lidocaine to line of skin incision and base of ilioinguinal nerve near anterior superior iliac spine; test sensation
2. Oblique **incision** extending from medial to the anterior superior iliac spine to pubis; incise Scarpa's fascia and expose external oblique fascia
3. Infiltrate 1% lidocaine beneath external oblique fascia (if local anesthesia); incise **external oblique** fascia in the direction of its fibers and extend *through* external ring; identify and protect ilioinguinal nerve
4. Bluntly separate **spermatic cord** from surrounding structures and encircle with a Penrose drain
5. Divide cremasteric fibers with sharp and blunt dissection, **free** hernia sac (anteromedial to cord for indirect) up to internal ring; open sac if indirect, and for either type reduce sac contents into abdomen (*beware* of sliding hernias)
6. For indirect hernia, ligate sac at its neck, and excise excess; for either type, **reduce** sac and secure in reduced position with Z-stitch
7. Cut polypropylene mesh to **fit** the contour of the inguinal floor, and create a slit to accommodate the spermatic cord as it exits the internal ring
8. Anchor inferior end of mesh to pubic tubercle, avoiding periostium (to decrease the risk of painful chronic osteitis); **suture** lateral/inferior edge of mesh to inguinal ligament and medial/superior edge to internal oblique aponeurosis with a nonabsorbable suture; the repair must be tension free
9. Suture overlapping tails of the mesh superior to the cord to create new **internal ring**
10. **Reapproximate** the edges of the external oblique fascia, and close incision in 2 layers with subcuticular suture or staples for skin; retract testis into scrotal sac

Risks/Results: Inguinal nerve injury, neuroma or neuritis, scrotal hematoma, testicular ischemia/loss, hernia recurrence, mesh infection

Hernia Repair, Inguinal — Laparoscopic (TAPP) [17]

Indications:

Selected patients with recurrent hernias or bilateral inguinal hernias

Setup: Position = supine and slight Trendelenberg; Foley

Procedure:

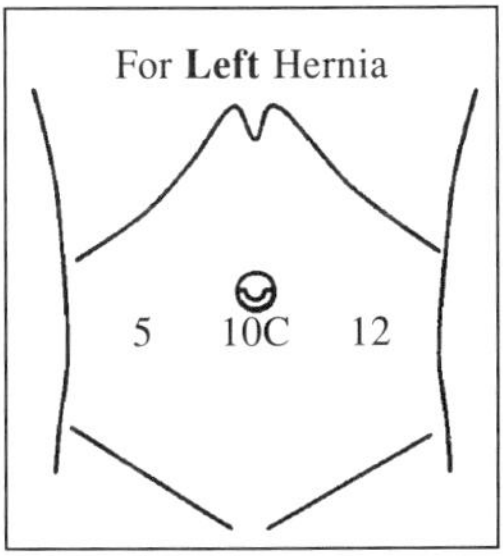

1. **Entry**: use umbilical incision to insert 10 mm Hasson trocar
2. Insert **12 mm port*** ~ 10 cm lateral to umbilicus on the side(s) of the hernia(s) under laparoscopic visualization (may be 5 mm port if 5 mm tacking device is used)
3. Insert a **5 mm port*** 10 cm lateral to umbilicus contralateral to the hernia defect(s) under laparoscopic visualization (*positions may be reversed)
4. **Incise peritoneum** transversely from medial umbilical ligament laterally past the lateral umbilical fold; bluntly dissect the peritoneal flap inferiorly, exposing the pre-peritoneal fat
5. **Reduce** any existing hernias
6. Bluntly dissect the **pre-peritoneal** fat, exposing Cooper's ligament, iliopubic tract, rectus abdominis fascia, and transversus abdominis fascia 2 cm above and lateral to internal ring.
7. Place nonabsorbable (e.g., polypropylene) **mesh** (± slit for cord) over Hesselbach's triangle and internal ring with the rounded side overlying the lateral edge of the rectus fascia
8. **Staple/tack** inferomedial portion of **mesh** to Cooper's ligament, proceed circumferentially, sequentially securing mesh to pubis, rectus fascia, and transversus abdominis fascia; do *not* staple the inferolateral edge of the mesh (*triangle of doom* containing iliac vessels; and lateral femoral cutaneous nerve)
9. **Reapproximate** peritoneal edges with staples
10. **Close** trocar sites > 5 mm either under direct vision or laparoscopically; close skin with subcuticular sutures, wound tapes

Risks: Hemorrhage, visceral injury (trocar related), mesh infection, nerve injury, recurrence

Hernia Repair, Umbilical (Open) [8]

Indications:

Adults: Any umbilical hernia should be repaired if the patient's medical condition permits
Children: 80 % of congenital umbilical hernias close by 2 years; if persistent, repair before school age

Setup: Position = supine

Procedure:

1. Make curvilinear infra-umbilical **incision**
2. **Dissect** subcutaneous tissue to expose hernia sac
3. **Free** the edges of the rectus fascia from sac
4. **Reduce** the sac into the abdominal cavity, or transect if adhesed to umbilicus (after confirming that nothing, or only omentum, lies within) and excise
5. If the defect is **small**, close primarily by approximating edges with one or more polypropylene sutures (simple interrupted, or figure-of-eight)
6. If the defect is **large**, separate rectus fascia from the underlying muscle on both sides and perform an imbricating closure; or use nonabsorbable mesh if necessary
7. Reapproximate **subcutaneous** tissues with absorbable sutures, and anchor umbilicus to fascia (avoid button-holing skin with stitch)
8. **Close** skin with running subcuticular absorbable sutures

Risks: Hemorrhage, bowel injury, infection, recurrence (rare in children)

Hernia Repair, Ventral/Incisional [18]

Indications:

Repair symptomatic hernias unless comorbid factors contraindicate intervention

Setup: Position = supine; consider NGT; foley

Procedure:

1. **Incise** skin over hernia defect and dissect tissue down to hernia sac
2. Free fascial edges surrounding sac of overlying fat until **healthy fascia** is identified
3. Separate the fascial edges from the hernia sac and **reduce** sac into abdomen
4. **Free** undersurface of fascia to expose strong, healthy fascia, and trim attenuated fascia
5. **Consider opening sac** if necessary to expose fascial edges; but protect underlying bowel by interposing omentum or peritoneum if plain/uncoated mesh is used
6. If facial edges can be approximated without tension, close fascia **primarily** with non-absorbable sutures
7. For larger hernias, cut nonabsorbable **prosthetic sheet** to size, at least 2 cm larger on all sides than defect
8. Use closely spaced horizontal mattress or simple interrupted sutures to **secure** prosthetic sheet to undersurface of fascia
9. **Consider** closed suction drain anterior to prosthetic sheet to prevent seroma/hematoma formation
10. **Close** subcutaneous tissue and skin

Postop: Abdominal binder for large hernia repairs, advance diet with return of bowel function

Risks: Wound or mesh infection (latter requiring mesh removal), bowel injury, hemorrhage, recurrence

Jejunostomy, Feeding — Open

Indications:

Enteral nutritional access in presence of proximal GI tract obstruction (e.g., due to neoplasm), gastroparesis or gastroesophageal reflux/aspiration

Setup: Position = supine; consider Foley, NGT

Procedure:

1. **Incision** as needed for concurrent procedure, otherwise small midline or transverse
2. Perform any **concurrent** procedures
3. **Select** loop of jejunum ~ 20–30 cm distal to LOT

Witzel

4. Insert feeding catheter through separate **stab wound** in anterior abdominal wall
5. **Insert catheter** distally through small incision into bowel lumen (antimesenteric), and secure with purse-string suture
6. Create ~ 5 cm proximal **tunnel** using interrupted seromuscular sutures
7. **Approximate** bowel to abdominal wall with seromuscular sutures
8. **Close** and secure catheter to skin with nonabsorbable suture

Needle-Catheter

4. Place **pursestring** suture at the bowel entrance site
5. Insert **trocar** through pursestring into bowel wall; tunnel sub-serosally for ~ 5 cm before entering lumen
6. **Thread feeding catheter** distally into lumen; create Witzel tunnel, as above (optional)
7. **Approximate** bowel to abdominal wall fascia with seromuscular sutures
8. **Close** and secure catheter to skin with nonabsorbable suture

Postop: Flush catheter *tid* (and after medications) to maintain patency; administer *only liquid* medications through tube; no medications should be given through needle-catheter J-tube

Risks: Hemorrhage, SBO, wound infection/dehiscence, tube dislodgment/erosion, peritonitis due to enteric/tube feed leakage into peritoneal cavity

Jejunostomy, Feeding — Laparoscopic [19]

Indications:

Enteral nutritional access in presence of proximal GI tract obstruction (e.g., due to neoplasm), gastroparesis or gastroesophageal reflux

Setup: Position = mild reverse Trendelenberg; Foley; NGT

Procedure:

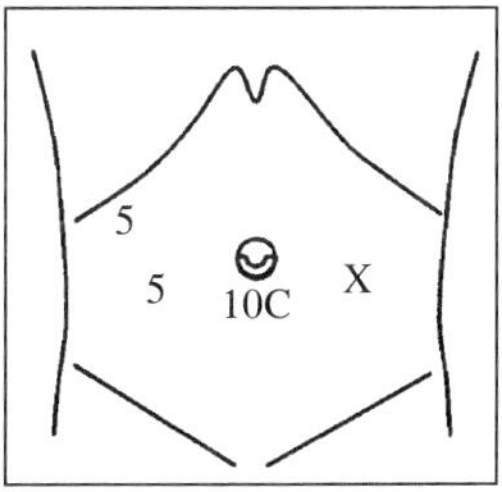

1. Open **Hasson** technique for placement of initial infraumbilical 10-mm camera port
2. **Insufflate** abdomen to ~ 10 mm Hg
3. Place two additional 5-mm **ports** to right of midline (See Figure)
4. Use graspers to **select loop** of jejunum 15-20 cm distal to LOT
5. Select abdominal wall tract site by **external palpation** in LUQ
6. **Approximate** bowel to abdominal wall with four transabdominally placed seromuscular sutures, leave loose or suture intracorporally
7. Insert 16-g **needle** through the abdominal wall (site marked "X") into the lumen of the bowel under direct visualization
8. Use **Seldinger** technique to dilate tract, then introduce feeding catheter distally into the jejunum
9. **Secure** transabdominal sutures over bolsters at the skin level; secure catheter with additional non-absorbable suture (alternatively, may secure jejunal loop to anterior abdominal wall at this point)
10. Remove ports and **close** incisions

Risks: Hemorrhage, SBO, wound infection/dehiscence, tube dislodgment/erosion, air embolus, trocar site hernia, peritonitis due to enteric/tube feed leakage into peritoneal cavity

Kidney Transplant [20-22]

Indications:

End-stage renal disease in a patient free of infection, deemed acceptable operative risk and candidate for life-long immunosupression

Setup: Position = supine; Foley, neosporin GU irrigant and clamp; NGT; A-line ± CVP/Swan depending on medical condition

Procedure:

1. Prepare graft on **back-table**: remove excessive fat, but do not devascularize ureter, leave Carrel patch (cuff) of donor aorta on renal artery if feasible
2. Keep kidney as **cool** as possible until arterial inflow is restored (e.g., w/ iced lap pads)
3. Preferably contralat to side of donor kidney, make curvilinear **skin incision** just superomedial to inguinal lig, divide/ligate inferior epigastrics and extend through muscle/fascial layers to enter preperitoneal space (do not violate peritoneum)
4. Gently **reflect** peritoneum and contents superomedially, place self-retaining retractor; sacrifice round lig., try to preserve spermatic cord by retracting laterally
5. **Expose/mobilize** iliac vessels generously
6. Clamp **external iliac vein** prox. and distally and perform end-to-side graft-external iliac vein anastomosis
7. Clamp **external iliac art.** prox. and distally and perform end-to-side graft-external iliac artery anastomosis
8. Distend bladder via Foley (then clamp), and incise serosa and muscle layers for 2–3 cm to create **submucosal tunnel**, spatulate distal donor ureter, and construct **ureteroneocystomy** (± over double-J stent), close bladder muscle over distal ureter
9. Ensure adequate **hemostasis**, consider closed suction drain(s) if hemostasis is marginal
10. **Position** kidney in iliac fossa pocket, **close** abdomen

Risks: Hemorrhage, injury to surrounding organs/spermatic cord, arterial or venous thrombosis, urine leak, lymphocele, wound or graft infection, wound dehiscence, opportunistic infection (e.g., fungal, CMV) or neoplasm due to immunosuppression, renal artery stenosis, ureteral stenosis, rejection (acute or chronic), direct side effects of immunosuppressive agents

Liver Transplant

Indications:

End-stage liver disease in a patient free of infection, deemed acceptable operative risk and candidate for life-long immunosupression

Setup: Foley, NGT, invasive monitoring; Position = supine, prep to include groins and axilla in the event that veno-venous bypass is required.

Procedure:

1. **Donor hepatectomy**, as described in "Organ Harvest" procedure
2. **Prepare** the donor liver by removing attached diaphragm, ligating phrenic veins, and right adrenal isolation; infuse UW solution and inspect for leaks
3. **Recipient hepatectomy**: Divide falciform, triangular, coronary, and gastrohepatic ligaments. Search for replaced left hepatic artery; divide cystic duct and artery, then left and right hepatic artery; mobilize portal vein, divide anterior pancreaticoduodenal branch, and divide portal vein near liver; divide adrenal vein. Isolate IVC and SVC enough to place a side-biting clamp on; remove liver. (Note: it may be necessary to use veno-venous bypass if the patient does not tolerate cross clamping the IVC; this is performed through catheters placed into the SVC via the L SC vein and the IVC via the left femoral vein.)
4. **Transplant**: Perform portal vein anastomosis end to end with 6-0 polypropylene, then hepatic artery anastomosis with 6-0 polypropylene (end-to-end or end-to-side); bile duct reconstruction end-to-end with 5-0 polypropylene (alternatively, perform end-to-side Roux-en-Y choledochojejunostomy); place 8 fr T-tube through separate incision in the CBD.
5. Perform open **feeding jejunostomy**
6. Place closed suction **drains** around anastomoses and **close** the abdomen

Risks: Bleeding, arterial or venous thrombosis, biliary anastomotic leak or stricture, rejection (acute or chronic), opportunistic infection, direct side effects of immunosuppressive agents

Lymph Node Dissection — Axillary [4]

Indications:

Staging and axillary control of breast cancer patients with or patients with melanoma or breast cancer who have a positive sentinel lymph node biopsy with drainage to axilla

Setup: Position = supine, arm extended; prep axilla, trunk and upper extremity

Procedure:

1. Make a transverse **incision** in the lower axilla, enter axillary fat pad, and develop circumferential skin flaps
2. **Retract** pectoralis major and pectoralis minor
3. **Identify** the axillary vein at the medial area of the pectoralis minor and begin ligating its tributaries with 3-0 silk; the anterior border of latissimus dorsi forms the lateral wall of the axilla, and the thoracodorsal nerve is found near the anterior border of latissimus dorsi (protect)
4. Working towards the medial wall of the axilla, **dissect** the lymph nodes and axillary fat together from the axilla
5. **Avoid** injuring the **long thoracic** nerve under the fascia of serratus anterior where the axillary vein passes over the second rib
6. Also **spare**, if possible, the following nerves: medial pectoral nerve, located superficial to the axillary vein and lateral to pectoralis minor; the lateral pectoral nerve, superficial to the axillary vein and medial to pectoralis minor; and the subscapular nerve in the vicinity of the subscapular artery and vein.
7. **Continue** dissection until specimen is separated from axillary vein and removed
8. **Mark** specimen with silk suture at superior aspect
9. **Drain** axillary cavity with 1-2 closed suction drains
10. **Close** subcutaneous tissue/deep dermis with interrupted, absorbable suture, and close skin with staples or subcuticular suture

Postop: Remove drains when drainage decreases (generally POD #4 or 5)

Risks: Bleeding, nerve injury (arm paresthesias, numbness, pain, winged scapula), lymphedema

Lymph Node Biopsy — Sentinel

Indications:

Intermediate thickness melanoma with no evidence of metastatic disease; stage I or II breast cancer

Setup: Position depends on location of primary tumor

Procedure:

1. Perform or schedule **lymphoscintigraphy** prior to surgery following injection of ^{99M}Tc sulfur colloid
2. In operating room, following the anesthetic, inject blue **dye** intradermally into 4–5 peritumoral sites using an insulin syringe, with a total volume of 1–2 ml; for breast tumors, may perform injection around non-palpable tumors intraparenchymally by U/S guidance, or subcutaneously or intradermally overlying the tumor.
3. Use hand-held gamma probe and films or skin markings made by the nuclear medicine team to guide the location of skin **incision** (2–3 cm length)
4. **Dissect** subcutaneous tissue using both blue afferent lymphatic channels and the hand-held gamma probe as guides to blue or radioactive lymph nodes; avoid injuring any blue-staining channels
5. **Remove** any **lymph nodes** with blue staining or radioactivity significantly greater than background levels and send to pathology (as sentinel lymph nodes; permanent ± frozen section)
6. Once all sentinel nodes are removed, **close** the subcutaneous tissue with interrupted absorbable sutures and the skin with a running subcuticular suture/steri-strips
7. Perform **formal lymph node dissection** if sentinel node(s) cannot be identified, or if sentinel node(s) + for tumor (practice still in evolution)

Risks: Failure to locate sentinel lymph node seen on preoperative lymphoscintigraphy; bleeding; infection

Melanoma Excision (Primary Tumor) [4]

Indications:

Definitive excision of biopsy-proven malignant melanoma after punch biopsy; re-excision with appropriate margins after excisional biopsy of small lesions

Setup: Position depends on location of primary tumor

Procedure:

1. **Placement** of incision should be along Langer's lines for maximum aesthetic closure and minimal tension
2. **Excise** the skin lesion and subcutaneous tissue with 1 cm radial margin for thin melanoma (< 1 mm) and 2 cm margin for all deeper lesions (*exception*: in areas, such as face/hands, where impact of wide margin on cosmesis or function is great, smaller margin is often necessary)
3. **Close** primarily if possible, although split-thickness skin grafts and flaps may be used if necessary
4. Regional **lymphadenectomy** is indicated for palpable lymphadenopathy but remains controversial in the absence of lymphadenopathy
5. **Sentinel lymph node mapping** should be considered for all intermediate thickness lesions, particularly when pathologic factors such as ulceration and regression are present, indicating a poorer prognosis

Postop: Monitor wound/skin graft for infection

Risks: Bleeding, infection, failed skin graft, local recurrence

Nissen Fundoplication — Laparoscopic [4,23,24]

Indications:

1. Symptomatic GERD refractory to medical management
2. In combination with repair of a large hiatal hernia
3. In combination with laparoscopic Heller myotomy for achalasia

Setup: Position monitors and assistants to provide clear lines of vision; pt = supine or modified lithotomy position depending on the preference of the operative surgeon to operate from between the patients legs or on the patient's right; NGT; IV antibiotics

Procedure:

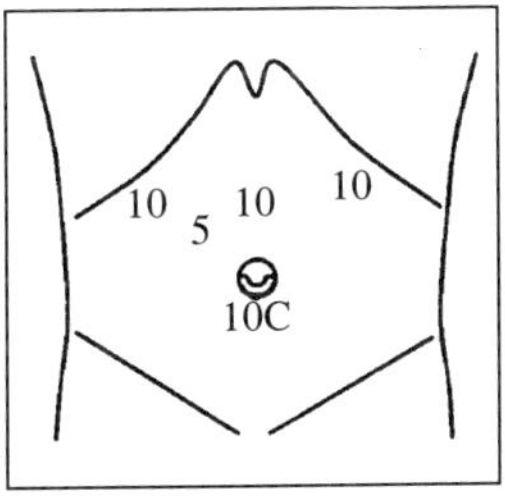

1. Midline 10 mm port at umbilicus or ~15 cm from xiphoid using open Hasson technique, create **pneumoperitoneum** to 15 mmHg and inspect abdomen
2. **Port placement** for instruments is variable depending on location of the surgeon (between legs or on right): insert two working ports in the upper abdomen under laparoscopic vision triangulating on the hiatus; insert an additional port in the left upper quadrant for placement of a laparoscopic Babcock clamp and an upper midline or right upper quadrant port for placement of liver (fan) retractor
3. Take down gastrohepatic ligament, identify **right crus**, and mobilize it from G-E junction; dissect behind the esophagus, staying above the epiphrenic fat pad
4. Identify the **left crus and** then encircle the esophagus with penrose drain, retract to the right, and complete the dissection of the left crus
5. If **reapproximation** of the crura is necessary, this is done with interrupted non-absorbable sutures
6. If necessary to mobilize the gastric fundus, divide the **short gastric** vessels with a Harmonic scalpel, linear cutting shears or clips
7. Pass **fundus** behind esophagus from left to right; if sufficiently mobilized the fundus should remain on the right without tension
8. With a 60 French bougie in esophagus, create 2.0 cm **wrap** with three seromuscular, interrupted sutures (pledgetted, if necessary) including bites of anterior esophageal wall
9. Wrap *may* be **secured** to the esophageal hiatus with interrupted sutures
10. Reexamine the entire abdomen, remove instruments under laparoscopic vision, and **close** port sites in a routine fashion

Risks: Hemorrhage, infection, injury to esophagus or bowel, pneumothorax, dysphagia, slipped wrap, port site hernia

Organ Procurement [6]

Indications:

To obtain donor organs (liver, pancreas, kidneys) for transplantation

Procedure:

1. **Incision**: midline laparotomy and median sternotomy
2. Mobilize left colon, right colon, and small bowel to identify and encircle the distal aorta; carry dissection superiorly on anterior surface of the aorta to the level of the left renal vein; **cannulate** distal **aorta**
3. Perform Kocher maneuver to identify and **isolate** infrarenal **IVC**
4. **Divide** inferior mesenteric vessels; identify and encircle bilateral distal ureters
5. Expose the **supraceliac aorta** in preparation for crossclamp, noting the presence of an aberrant left hepatic artery (20 % of donors)
6. **Preparation of Liver**: Begin dissection of the porta hepatis at the common hepatic artery; note the presence of an aberrant right hepatic artery (13% of donors) by palpation; divide the distal CBD and flush the duct of bile via an incision in the gallbladder; identify and cannulate the SMV or portal vein for portal cooling and perfusion of preservative solution.
7. **Preparation of Pancreas**: Divide the gastrocolic ligament, gastrosplenic, and lienophrenic ligaments to provide complete mobilization of the spleen which is used as a handle to aid in the left to right dissection of the pancreas from its retroperitoneal attachments; ligate and divide the small bowel mesenteric root caudal to the pancreas
8. **Cooling Procedure**: With cardioplegic arrest, begin perfusion of preservative solution via the distal aortic cannula (2 L) and the portal cannula (2 L), crossclamp supraceliac aorta, and pour slushed saline into the abdominal cavity for topical cooling; monitor cooling by palpation and inspection of organs; vent preservative fluid to right chest via incision in supradiaphragmatic cava or pulmonary veins
9. **Organ extraction**: **Liver** — divide the triangular attachments to the diaphragm, divide the aorta at the supraceliac clamp and at the level of the SMA, divide the suprahepatic IVC with a cuff of diaphragm, divide the infrahepatic IVC above the renal veins, and divide the portal vein; **pancreas** — divide the proximal peripancreatic duodenum and proximal jejunum with stapler and remove pancreas with its arterial supply; **kidneys** — mobilize and divide the distal ureters and dissect the renal structures from their posterior attachments, remove the kidneys with cuffs of perirenal IVC and aorta
10. Procure donor distal aorta, iliac arteries, and iliac veins for **vessel conduits.**

Pancreas Transplantation (with Enteric Drainage) [26,27]

Indications:

Brittle diabetes, hypoglycemic unawareness, early diabetic nephropathy, and diabetes with functioning kidney transplants

Setup:

Preoperative bowel preparation
Anesthesia = General
Position = Supine; Foley, ECG, oximetry, A-line

Procedure:

1. **Enter** abdomen through a generous midline incision.
2. Skeletonize **common iliac** (CI) vessels from surrounding tissue.
3. **Ligate lymphatics** to prevent postoperative lymphocele.
4. Obtain proximal and distal **control** of **CI vein**
5. Bring **donor pancreas** onto table
6. Perform end-to-side **anastomosis** between donor portal vein and recipient **CI vein**
7. Perform end-to side **anastomosis** between donor iliac Y-graft and recipient **CI artery** and sequentially release vascular clamps
8. Pick a segment of jejunum 30–40 cm from the ligament of Treitz and perform a side-of-donor duodenum to side-of-recipient jejunum anastomosis (**enteric drainage**)
9. Assure **hemostasis** with 3-0 silk sutures and electrocautery
10. Irrigate abdomen and **close** fascia with a running nonabsorbable suture

Risks/Results: Major 3–8%: Venous thrombosis (within 1st 24 hrs), hemorrhage, enteric anastomotic leak, intraabdominal abscess, wound infection, graft rejection, operative mortality (2–3%); one-year graft survival 50–60%

Pancreatic Cystogastrostomy/-jejunostomy

Indications:

Symptomatic pancreatic pseudocyst present for greater than 6 weeks, without indications of malignancy

Setup: Supine, NGT, foley, GET anesthesia

Procedure:

1. Midline or left subcostal **incision**
2. **Identify** pseudocyst
3. **Assess** accessibility to stomach for possible cyst-gastrostomy; if this is not possible, a loop of jejunum may be brought up as a Roux-en-Y to drain the cyst
4. **Open** the cyst, send excised portion of cyst wall to pathology as the **biopsy**
5. Construct an **anastomosis** to the stomach or jejunum using interrupted absorbable sutures or stapler
6. Place **drains** around anastomosis
7. Consider **feeding jejunostomy** based on nutritional status (not usually indicated)
8. **Close** abdomen

Risks: Bleeding, pancreatic anastomotic leak/fistula, wound infection/dehiscence, septic complications

Pancreatectomy, Distal [4,8]

Indications:

***Urgent*:** Trauma
***Elective*:** Neoplasm, chronic pancreatitis/pseudocyst, cyst

Setup: Position = supine; Foley; NGT; ± A-line

Procedure:

1. Perform midline or subcostal **incision**
2. **Explore** abdomen
3. **Enter** lesser sac through gastrocolic ligament, reflect left colon inferiorly
4. **Incise** peritoneum inferior and superior to pancreas; come around pancreas with finger
5. Mobilize spleen; complete **dissection** of body and tail of pancreas
6. Identify **splenic artery** and doubly **ligate**; ligate short gastric and left gastroepiploic arteries
7. Gently free **splenic vein** from pancreas and **ligate** (alternatively, ligate in next step if cutting stapler is used to transect pancreas)
8. **Transect** pancreas, remove pancreatic tail and spleen; place row of interrupted 00 silk polypropylene or absorbable monofilament sutures in a mattress fashion entirely through pancreas
9. Place closed suction **drain** near pancreatic stump
10. Irrigate and **close**

Postop: NGT for gastric decompression

Risks: Hemorrhage, pancreatic leak/fistula, abscess, MI, pneumonia, SBO, wound infection/dehiscence

Pancreaticoduodenectomy (Whipple Procedure)

Indications:

Resectable mass in the head of the pancreas without evidence of lymphatic or metastatic spread of tumor

Setup: Light preop bowel preparation; Position = Supine; NGT, foley, GET anesthesia

Procedure:

1. Bilateral subcostal **incision, explore** abdomen for metastatic disease (peritoneal surfaces/underside of diaphragm, omentum, liver, hepatoduodenal ligament, celiac nodes)
2. **Exposure**: place self-retaining retractor, and pack intestines away from pancreaticoduodenal complex, retract omentum superiorly and open lesser sac
3. Perform **cholecystectomy**
4. Remove omentum from distal stomach, place clamps across distal stomach (antral-sparing approach) or just distal to pylorus (pylorus-sparing), and **divide stomach** sharply or with cautery, or using a stapler
5. Perform generous **Kocher** maneuver, mobilize head of pancreas/duodenum complex, **divide common bile duct** sharply, and temporarily occlude the proximal end
6. **Palpate head** of pancreas to confirm mass; *may* biopsy mass transduodenally if biopsy results will affect management (not routinely necessary); palpate **neck** of pancreas between left thumb and forefinger — if tumor *prohibits* clean separation of portal vein and SMA (particularly latter) from pancreas, the tumor is typically deemed unresectable, warranting abortion of resection (and performance of biliary bypass and/or gastrojejunostomy instead)
7. Take gastroduodenal artery, **divide pancreatic neck** with electrocautery, divide remaining soft tissue/uncinate process with stapler or between clamps, suture ligate major vessels
8. Mobilize duodenum to proximal jejunum, take down ligament of Treitz, **divide distal duodenum** or proximal jejunum near ligament of Treitz with linear cutting stapler, divide **uncinate**, complete mobilization of specimen and **remove**
9. **Reconstruct** with Roux jejunal limb to pancreatic duct using duct-to-mucosa end-to-end or end-to-side anastomosis (single-layer or two-layer), to CBD end-to-side (single-layer), and to stomach end-to-side (double-layer, retrocolic)
10. Place closed suction **drains, close** abdomen

Risks: Hemorrhage, pancreatitis, anastomotic leak/fistula, abscess, MI, pneumonia, SBO, wound infection/dehiscence

Pancreaticojejunostomy, Lateral (Puestow) [8]

Indications:

Chronic pancreatitis with dilated main pancreatic duct, refractory to medical management

Setup: Position = supine; Foley; NGT; ± A-line

Procedure:

1. Perform bilateral subcostal (Chevron) or long midline **incision**; **explore** abdomen for ulceration, stones, malignancy
2. Free and retract the omentum and stomach to **expose** the entire length of pancreas
3. **Identify** the pancreatic duct (PD) by needle aspiration, examine for stones
4. **Incise PD** for 6-8 cm to the right (stopping before reaching GDA medially)
5. **Clear** the duct of stones
6. Divide jejunum ~ 15-20 cm distal to LOT; pass distal arm through defect in transverse mesocolon (**roux-en-Y**)
7. **Divide** the open end of the arm along its antimesenteric border for a length slightly greater than the PD incision
8. Perform single-layer **anastomosis** of entire wall of jejunum to capsule of pancreas with 3-0 or 4-0 absorbable suture; close or anastomose the open end of the jejunum
9. Perform end-to-side **anastomosis** of the proximal arm of the divided jejunum to a loop of jejunum distal to the pancreaticojejunostomy
10. Consider feeding jejunostomy if severe malnutrition; irrigate and **close**

Postop: NGT for gastric decompression; resume pancreatic enzyme therapy when taking po's

Risks: Hemorrhage, pancreatitis, anastomotic leak/fistula, abscess, MI, pneumonia, SBO, wound infection/dehiscence

Parathyroidectomy

Indications:

Primary, secondary, or tertiary hyperparathyroidism unresponsive to medical therapy. Localizing studies are controversial. Multiple endocrine neoplasia syndromes should be investigated preoperatively.

Setup: Supine with neck extended, GET anesthesia

Procedure:

1. Low collar skin **incision** above the sternal notch
2. **Transect** platysma
3. **Separate** strap muscles at midline
4. Free up right or left thyroid lobe being careful to **identify/preserve** recurrent laryngeal nerve and identify right upper and lower parathyroid glands.
5. **Divide** middle thyroid vein to increase exposure
6. To assure the presence of parathyroid tissue, send each gland to pathology for **frozen** section; alternatively, when available, parathyroid hormone rapid assays are performed to assure removal of appropriate tissue.
7. If there is one **dominant adenoma**, this may be removed in isolation. For **MEN I** patient or renal failure patients, either 3.5 glands are removed, or 4 glands are removed, with reimplantation of part of one gland into the sternocleidomastoid muscle or forearm.

Postop: Check calcium level; observe for signs of hypocalcemia or stridor/respiratory difficulties from hematoma formation in the neck

Risks: Permanent hypoparathyroidism/hypocalcemia, recurrent laryngeal nerve injury, hematoma formation with potential for airway compromise

Peritoneal Dialysis Catheter Placement [28-30]

Indications:

CAPD for chronic renal failure in the following settings: poor vascular access options, repeated infections of vascular access sites, critical or poor medical condition, small children, AIDS, coagulopathy, pt preference (for CAPD)
Short-term peritoneal dialysis in patients with ARF, with CRF who become temporarily dialysis-dependent, or requiring temporary dialysis access while hemodialysis access matures, or for core rewarming in severe hypothermia

Contraindications: Peritonitis, peritoneal soilage, dense adhesions, respiratory insufficiency, peritoneal malignancy, large ventral hernia, lack of diaphragmatic integrity

Setup: Position = supine; enema prior to OR, foley catheter (if pt makes urine); have saline and arterial (valveless) pressure tubing available in OR

Procedure:

1. Make 2 cm **infraumbilical** incision, dissect through fascia, and make a small incision in the peritoneum
2. **Inspect** the abdomen for adhesions (use a laparoscope if necessary)
3. Load the PD catheter on a stilette, **insert** through fascia on either side of incision and into the abdominal cavity, aiming for the pelvis (laparoscopy may be used to aid in positioning of the catheter)
4. Remove the stilette and **confirm** function of the catheter by instilling 500 cc of saline via valveless tubing, insuring free forward and return flow
5. Make 0.5 cm **counter-incision** lateral to the umbilicus (also, avoid belt line)
6. **Tunnel** the extraperitoneal end of the catheter to the exit site, positioning one Dacron cuff at the peritoneum and one at least 2 cm from the skin exit site in the subcutaneous tract (if one cuff, position anterior to rectus sheath within subQ)
7. Place a **pursestring** suture around the internal Dacron cuff of the catheter at the peritoneum ensuring a water tight seal
8. **Close** the rectus fascia and skin in a routine fashion
9. **Confirm** continued free flow of dialysate through catheter with no evidence of leak
10. **Secure** the catheter at exit site, dress wounds, cap catheter

Postop: Catheter should be allowed to mature for 1–2 weeks to insure wound healing has created a water tight seal around catheter; if necessary, PD may be initiated shortly after procedure provided the patient remains in a supine position during dwells

Risks/Results: Hemorrhage, injury to bowel or other viscus, catheter leakage or malfunction (2-year patency 50–60%), wound infection, peritonitis (including candidal/fungal), small bowel obstruction, ileus

Small Bowel Resection [4,8]

Indications:

Urgent: Small bowel gangrene/perforation, GI bleeding of small bowel origin
Elective: Small bowel neoplasm, inflammatory bowel disease refractory to medical Rx

Setup: Position = supine; Foley, NGT

Procedure:

1. **Midline abdominal incision**
2. **Relieve obstruction**, if present, through lysis of adhesions, reduction of hernia
3. **Determine viability** considering color, odor, pulse, Doppler signal, fluorescein-Wood's lamp test, carefully **eviscerate** involved bowel from peritoneal cavity
4. **Divide** bowel between clamps on each side of lesion; angle clamps to preserve anti-mesenteric blood supply
5. **Ligate** and divide mesentery close to bowel (unless malignancy); remove specimen
6. **Confirm viability** of remaining bowel
7. Perform stapled functional end-to-end **anastomosis** (*check* mucosal aspect of staple line for *bleeding*, place figure-of-eight sutures to address any bleeding sites), *OR* hand-sewn single- or double-layer end-to-end anastomosis (side-to-side if marked size discrepancy)
8. **Close** mesenteric **defect** with 3-0 chromic
9. **Assess patency** of anastomosis by palpating between thumb and forefinger and estimating size of lumen
10. **CLOSE**: Irrigate; consider retention sutures if pt is on steroids, diabetic, or poorly nourished; close wound

Risks: Hemorrhage, wound infection/dehiscence, anastomotic leak

Splenectomy — Open [4,8]

Indications:

***Emergent*:** Trauma
***Elective*:** Treatment of hypersplenism (primary, or secondary to ITP/hematologic disorders or other processes), diagnosis, staging (e.g., Hodgkin's disease), splenic abscess

Setup: Position = supine; Foley; NGT

Procedure:

1. Perform **left subcostal** incision or midline incision for trauma
2. **Explore** LUQ and abdomen for accessory splenic tissue (e.g., splenic hilum, omentum)
3. Divide **gastrosplenic** ligament/short gastric vessels
4. Identify **splenic artery**, dissect artery and ligate with silk suture if well exposed at this point (optional)
5. Deliver spleen into wound and divide **splenorenal ligament**
6. Identify and divide **splenocolic** and **splenophrenic ligaments**
7. Identify and divide **splenic vein** and **splenic artery** (if not ligated previously)
8. **Remove** spleen
9. Irrigate, confirm **hemostasis**
10. **Close**

Postop: Pneumovax and H flu vaccine either preop or 4–5 days postop; consider NGT

Risks: Hemorrhage, pancreatitis, post-splenectomy sepsis, wound infection/dehiscence

Splenectomy — Laparoscopic

Indications:

Elective: Treatment of hypersplenism (primary, or secondary to ITP/hematologic disorders or other processes), diagnosis, staging (e.g., Hodgkin's disease), splenic abscess

Setup: Position = supine; Foley; NGT

Procedure:

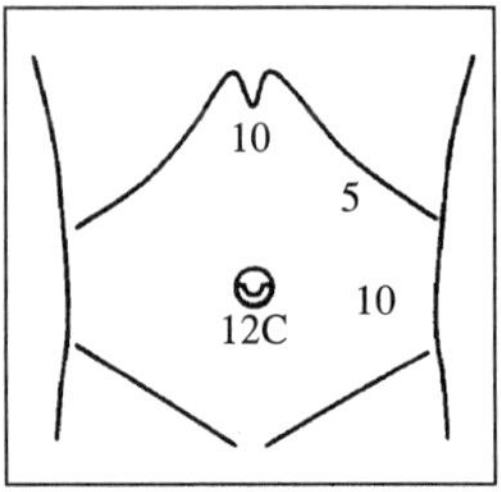

1. Vertical or transverse supra- or infraumbilical 1–2 cm **incision**, incise fascia (vertically) and place traction sutures through each side of fascia
2. Enter fascia/peritoneum under direct visualization with Hasson trocar and insufflate with CO_2 to 15 mm Hg (open technique) to create **pneumoperitoneum**
3. Introduce **laparoscope**, place pt in reverse Trendelenberg position and airplane to the left, place trocars as shown, explore for accessory splenic tissue (e.g., splenic hilum, omentum) or other pathology
4. **Transect short gastric vessels** (with clips or ultrasonic dissector)
5. **Transect splenic artery** (with vascular load of stapler, clips, or ties)
6. Divide **splenocolic, splenorenal, and splenophrenic ligaments**
7. Identify **splenic vein** (and artery, if not ligated previously), divide with stapler, clips or ties
8. **Remove** spleen by placing in endoscopic retrieval bag and morcellating through a large port site (caution: do not allow spillage of splenic fragments into peritoneal cavity)
9. Irrigate, confirm **hemostasis**
10. **Close**

Postop: Pneumovax and H flu vaccine either preop or 4–5 days post-op; consider NGT

Risks: Hemorrhage, pancreatitis, post-splenectomy sepsis, wound infection, air embolus, trocar site hernia

Thyroidectomy [4,8]

Indications:

Neoplasm, symptomatic goiter, hyperthyroidism

Setup: Position = supine with neck extended

Procedure:

1. Perform transverse, **low cervical** incision
2. Elevate **flaps** to notch of thyroid cartilage and jugular notch
3. Elevate and retract **strap** muscles
4. Bluntly **dissect** the thyroid gland laterally; retract the lobe(s) medially and anteriorly for excision
5. **Ligate** middle thyroid vein
6. **Identify** recurrent laryngeal nerve by blunt dissection in the tracheoesophageal groove; identify and protect parathyroid glands
7. Identify and **ligate** inferior thyroid artery and lower pole vessels; ligate the superior thyroid artery and upper pole vessels
8. Dissect the lobe(s) from the trachea by **dividing** the gland between straight clamps; minimum resection for confirmed malignancy is lobectomy + isthmusectomy
9. Suture **ligate** the thyroid on the trachea and isthmus
10. **Close**

Postop: √ Calcium, thyroid function

Risks: Hemorrhage, thyroid storm, hypoparathyroidism, recurrent laryngeal nerve injury, wound infection, hematoma, potential airway compromise

Tracheostomy [4,31]

Indications:

Ventilator dependence; slow/difficult ventilator weaning; upper airway obstruction; for control of secretions

Setup: Position = semi-Fowler position; hyperextend neck (if no C-spine fracture); place towel roll beneath shoulders; support head with donut-shaped cushion

Procedure:

1. Transverse cervical **incision** 2 finger-breadths above sternal notch
2. **Dissect** down in midline between strap muscles to locate trachea
3. Retract thyroid **isthmus** superiorly or clamp and divide it
4. Expose and clean anterior surface of **trachea**; locate 2nd–3rd rings
5. Place **stay sutures** around tracheal rings and use to elevate and immobilize trachea (*avoid* puncturing endotracheal tube balloon with needle)
6. When ready, **notify** anesthesiology personnel to pull endotracheal tube back above level of incision in order to avoid puncturing balloon of ET tube
7. Make a trap-door shaped **incision** or vertical incision through the 2nd–3rd rings (do not incise the first ring) of trachea
8. Enlarge the opening with a tracheal spreader and place **tracheostomy tube** inside trachea as endotracheal tube is backed out
9. **Attach** ventilator tubing to tracheostomy tube
10. **Anchor** each corner of tracheostomy tube to skin with silk sutures and secure tracheostomy tube with umbilical tape or velcro fastener placed around patient's neck

Postop: Monitor tracheostomy site closely for bleeding during immediate postop period

Risks: Bleeding, loss of airway control, tracheo-innominate fistula, esophageal injury, tracheoesophageal fistula, tracheal stenosis

Trauma Laparotomy [32-34]

Indications:

Penetrating trauma with possible or proven penetration of fascia or intra-abd injury
Blunt: unstable blunt abd trauma pt with + DPL or abd U/S, or unknown source of hypotension; blunt abd trauma pt with indication for sgy on plain films or CT scan, or initially stable pt with liver/spleen injury who fails observation; pt with peritonitis

Setup: Position = supine; IV access (= 2 lg.-bore IVs ± cordis); A-line ± CVP line; Foley; NGT; prep from chin to ankles (provide access to groins for CPB and at least one ankle for saphenous vein graft); PRBC avail.; 2 suction apparati, cautery setups, etc.

Procedure:

1. Generous **midline** abd incision (possible exceptions: graze wound, small children), use Mayo scissors (not cautery) for fascia
2. Rapidly **evacuate** blood, clots, and if necessary occlude aorta beneath diaphragm (manually may be fastest, then with aortic occluder against vertebral column, then with aortic clamp if this can be achieved quickly and safely)
3. **Pack** all four quadrants of abd with lap pads, remove sequentially and inspect for sources of bleeding from major vessels and/or organs (e.g., aorta, IVC, liver, pelvic vessels), compress; proximal and distal control
4. Control hemorrhage from **vessels** using direct pressure with fingers, spongestick, lap pad, or with intraluminal application of Foley or Fogarty catheter; obtain prox/distal control and quickly repair or ligate sources of major bleeding
5. Control hemorrhage from **organs** (e.g., liver, spleen, pancreas, kidney) with packing and/or direct pressure; liver hemorrhage may require porta hepatis occlusion (Pringle) ± supra- and infrahepatic caval occlusion
6. After gross hemorrhage control, prevent further **soilage** from GI perforations using clamp (e.g., Babcock) and/or stapler
7. **Explore** central retroperitoneal hematomas by medial visceral rotation: left (Mattox) exposes upper abd aorta, right (Cattel) exposes infrahepatic IVC; explore selected perirenal hematomas (e.g., expanding, nonperfused on IVP or etc.) after renal vascular pedicle control (controversial)
8. Thoroughly **survey** abdomen: examine all four quadrants, all peritoneal surfaces, diaphragm, liver/biliary tract, lesser sac/pancreas, spleen, stomach/duodenum, run small bowel starting from LOT, large bowel, GU system

9. **Repair** appropriate injuries, resect/repair/divert bowel as necessary if pt can tolerate
10. Consider placement of feeding G- or J-tube, and **close** abdomen (may necessitate silo or other temporary closure in case of damage control or inability to close primarily)

Risks: Hemorrhage, coagulopathy, sepsis, renal failure, pneumonia, MODS, SBO, wound infection/dehiscence, missed injury (e.g., SB), abdominal compartment syndrome

Section 2
VASCULAR SURGERY

AAA Repair [35]

Indications:

Emergent: Ruptured/leaking AAA
Urgent: Symptomatic or mycotic AAA
Elective: AAA diam > 5 cm; or > 4 cm with rapid enlargement (> 0.5 cm/6 mos) in patient with life expectancy of ≥ 2 years

Setup: Position = Supine (for transabd); Foley; NGT; A-line± CVP/Swan; ± cell-saver

Procedure (Unruptured):

1. Generous **midline** abd incision, and **explore** abd (e.g., neoplasms)
2. Self-retaining **retractor**
3. **Exposure**: retract small bowel to left, reflect transverse colon superiorly to expose D4 and ligament of Treitz
4. Make generous vertical incision in **peritoneum** over aneurysm, identify left renal vein (courses *post*eriorly ~ 5% of cases) and retract superiorly
5. **Dissect** aorta proximally and laterally, iliac arteries if bifurcated graft
6. Administer **heparin** ~ 100 units/kg IV
7. Alert anesthesia: **clamp** aorta proximally, then distally (iliac aa if bifurc graft)
8. **Incise aneurysm** vertically, remove clot, irrigate, ligate lumbars and IMA (reimplant IMA into graft if large, is only patent visceral vessel, or sigmoid dusky after ligation)
9. Prox **anastomosis**, clamp graft, then distal anastomosis; irrigate, flush clot/debris out by slowly releasing proximal clamp prior to tying final distal anastomotic suture, then open flow to internal iliacs (flush debris), then to external iliacs/lower extremities
10. Close sac over graft, close posterior peritoneum, reassess rectosigmoid viability, **close** abdomen

Risks: Hemorrhage, MI, ARF, pneumonia, rectosigmoid ischemia or infarction, LE ischemia, distal embolization/trash toe, paraplegia, SBO, wound infection/dehiscence, graft infection, anastomotic leak/rupture, groin infection or lymphocele (for bifurcated graft), impotence, aortoenteric fistula

Amputation — Above-Knee [8,36]

Indications:

Lower extremity gangrene in nonambulatory pt, or when below-knee amputation is not feasible or fails to heal; neoplasm or trauma rendering limb unsalvageable

Contraindications:

Potential for limb salvage with potential benefit to patient

Setup: Position = supine with ipsilateral leg abducted and elevated; consider tourniquet; Anesthesia = general or low spinal

Procedure:

1. **Incise** skin circumferentially with equal anterior and posterior flaps (fishmouth); flaps should be as long as is feasible
2. Incise subcutaneous tissue, divide/ligate greater saphenous vein, and divide fascia and **anterior** muscle bellies
3. Divide femoral **vessels** between clamps
4. Divide/ligate femoral **nerve**, and allow to retract
5. Clear periosteum off **femur** and divide with saw
6. Sharply divide **posterior** muscle bellies in line with skin incision
7. Complete posterior **flap**
8. Irrigate wound and ensure **hemostasis** (observing closely for several minutes after releasing tourniquet, if used)
9. **Reapproximate** anterior and posterior edges of investing fascia with interrupted absorbable sutures, close skin with staples or nonabsorbable monofilament sutures
10. Dress with layer of Vaseline gauze against suture line, then sterile gauze, and soft **dressing**

Postop Care:

Elevate limb postop
Remove dressing on POD 4–5
Initiate physical therapy
Remove skin sutures after several weeks, depending on steroid use/nutritional status

Risks: Hemorrhage, skin necrosis or failure of wound healing, wound infection, MI

Amputation — Below-Knee [8,36]

Indications:

Gangrene; failure of limb-salvage bypass procedure; neoplasm or trauma rendering distal limb unsalvageable

Setup: Position = supine w/ ipsilat. leg abducted, elevated; ± tourniquet; aim to divide tibia at least 8–10 cm distal to tibial tuberosity

Procedure:

1. **Incise** skin circumferentially: (1) long posterior flap or (2) equal anterior and posterior flaps (fishmouth)
2. Incise subcutaneous tissue, fascia and divide **anterior muscle** bellies
3. Divide anterior tibial **neurovascular** bundle between clamps
4. Divide **fibula** 2–3 cm proximal to planned line of division of tibia using double-action bone cutters
5. Clear periosteum off **tibia and** divide with saw, beveling anterior lip superiorly
6. Divide **posterior** muscle bellies in line with skin incision, dividing remaining posterior tibial and peroneal neurovascular bundles between clamps
7. **File** anterior edge of tibia to minimize risk of pressure necrosis of overlying skin
8. Irrigate wound and ensure **hemostasis** (observe closely for several minutes after releasing tourniquet, if used)
9. **Reapproximate** anterior and posterior edges of investing fascia with interrupted absorbable sutures, close skin with staples or nonabsorbable monofilament sutures
10. Dress with layer of Vaseline gauze against suture line, then sterile gauze, and plaster splint, or equivalent **dressing** to stabilize limb in slight flexion, followed by stockingette; avoid over-tightening dressing, which results in skin ischemia and necrosis

Postop:

Immobilize (to prevent contractures) and elevate limb
Remove dressing on POD 4–5
Initiate physical therapy with active ROM exercises upon removal of dressing
Remove skin sutures at several weeks, dependent upon steroid use and nutritional status

Risks: Hemorrhage, skin necrosis or failure of wound healing, wound infection, MI

Amputation — Transmetatarsal [8,36]

Indications:

Gangrene of ≥ 2 toes with warm foot, adequate blood supply for healing; chronic osteomyelitis of toes

Setup: Position = supine, ipsilateral leg elevated

Procedure:

1. Make midtarsal transverse **incision** through skin and subQ across dorsum of foot, angling slightly toward heel at corners to avoid dog-ears
2. **Extend** incision longitudinally starting from lateral or medial side, and curve transversely near proximal toe crease to create long posterior flap (final incision appears like an "L" when left foot viewed from the side)
3. Expose and divide **metatarsals** sequentially with bone cutters, debride with rongeurs if needed
4. Divide **tendons**, and allow to retract
5. Irrigate and ensure **hemostasis**
6. Cover wound with flap, and approximate **fascia** with interrupted absorbable sutures
7. Reapproximate **skin** with staples or nonabsorbable sutures
8. Apply Vaseline or betadine gauze over wound followed by dry gauze **dressing**

Postop: Change dressing on POD 4 or 5, then touch-down weight-bearing with physical therapy

Follow-up:

Remove skin sutures at 3–4 weeks
Physical therapy, Orthotics

Risks: Hemorrhage, skin necrosis or failure of wound healing, wound infection

Aortofemoral Bypass [8]

Indications:

Disabling claudication (or LeRiche Syndrome) in an acceptable operative candidate
Critical limb ischemia — tissue necrosis, rest pain (rare in the absence of distal disease)
Atheroembolism — blue toe syndrome from ulcerated plaques in atherosclerotic aorta

Setup: Position = supine, prep from nipples to ankles

Procedure:

1. Expose femoral sheath through vertical femoral incision, and isolate common, superficial, and profunda **femoral arteries** bilaterally
2. **Open** abdomen in midline from xyphoid to pubis, and pack intestines into right upper quadrant, place self-retaining retractor
3. Incise retroperitoneum and **expose aorta** from renal vein to inferior mesenteric artery
4. Administer IV **heparin**
5. Notify anesthesia, cross **clamp** aorta both proximal and distal to site of anastomosis; choice of anastomosis: end-to-end, or end-to-side (latter is preferred in presence of complete external iliac occlusions since it preserves hypogastric perfusion)
6. Divide (for end-to-end) or incise (end-to-side) aorta between proximal and distal clamps; **proximal** graft **anastomosis** using running polypropylene suture (2-0 to 4-0) starting with the posterior wall of the aorta, running both arms, and securing suture line anteriorly
7. Clamp graft, release proximal aortic clamp, **check** suture line for bleeding/patency
8. **Tunnel** limbs of graft to femoral incisions; **clamp** common, superficial, and profunda femoral arteries
9. For each side, make arteriotomy over distal common femoral artery; perform end-to-side **femoral** artery **anastomoses** using running 5-0 polypropylene sutures starting proximally; release proximal graft clamp and flush air out of limbs prior to securing suture line (restore flow to one leg while performing 2nd distal anastomosis)
10. **Close** retroperitoneum over graft, close fascia, abdominal wall, and inguinal incisions

Postop: Check neurovascular exam regularly, monitor in ICU

Risks: MI, bleeding, thrombosis, intestinal ischemia, atheroembolism, compartment syndrome

Axillobifemoral Bypass

Indications:

Urgent/Emergent: Mycotic abdominal aortic aneurysm; aortoduodenal fistula, infected aortic graft.
Elective: disabling claudication, rest pn, gangrene or ulceration in presence of high-grade stenosis/occlusion of aortoiliac system esp. high risk patients: elderly, severe cardiopulmonary dz, hostile abdomen; provide inflow for infrainguinal bypass procedures in high-risk patients with combined aortoiliac and femoropopliteal disease

Setup: **Anesthesia**: General or combination of epidural and local with heavy sedation during tunneling. **Position**: Supine with (operative side) arm abducted 90º, Foley, ECG, oximetry, A-line, CVP line, PA catheter for high-risk cardiac pts; prep right axilla and groins prior to incision particularly in the obese; prep skin widely from supraclavicular area to thighs bilaterally

Procedure: (Consider two-team approach)

1. Perform **femorofemoral** bypass as described in fem-fem section
2. Make infraclavicular **incision**, two finger breadths below midportion of right clavicle
3. Bluntly separate fibers of P. major and mobilize and retract P. minor laterally; and mobilize and retract axillary vein inferiorly; **mobilize axillary artery** medial to thoracoacromial artery
4. Create **tunnel** between right groin incision and axillary incision, passing medial to the ASIS to the midaxillary line, and then posterior to P. major into axilla.
5. **Pass** 8 mm ringed PTFE **graft** through tunnel
6. Obtain **proximal and distal control** on axillary artery, CFA and Fem-Fem graft, administer **heparin** 100 U/kg
7. Perform **proximal anastomosis** side-to-end on axillary artery, routing graft parallel to axillary artery for 8-10 cm
8. Perform **distal anastomosis** end-to-side to fem-fem graft at its anastomosis with the right CFA
9. **Assess** ankle/foot vascular status (with doppler if necessary), selective completion arteriography for complicated or technically problematic procedures
10. Ensure **hemostasis**, **close** in 2 to 3 layers

PostOp: ASA 81 or 325mg QD. Clinic 2 wks postop to √Sx, wound, pulses, ABI. Q3 months for ABI and duplex scanning. Q6 month F/U √Sx, pulses in feet and grafts.

Risks/Results: Local hemorrhage, proximal graft disruption (1–5%), acute thrombosis, MI, stroke, pneumonia, DVT/PE, upper extremity thromboembolism, wound infection/dehiscence, graft infection (1.5%), perigraft seroma, pseuodaneurysm. 5yr primary patency 35–75%; 5yr survival 50%

Carotid Endarterectomy [8]

Indications:

TIA(s) or completed stroke (following recovery) in distribution of carotid stenosis (>60%); asymptomatic carotid stenosis > 80–90% (selected patients with > 70% stenosis)

Setup: Position = supine, with head extended and turned toward contralateral side; **OPTIONS** to ensure adequacy of collateral flow during the procedure: a) perfusion shunt; b) intraop EEG; c) clinical exam if performed under MAC

Procedure:

1. **Incise** skin over anterior border of SCM, retract muscle laterally, avoid injury to facial, hypoglossal, and greater auricular nerves
2. Divide **facial vein** anterior to carotid sheath — consider harvesting facial vein (alt., ext. carotid or saphenous vein) if vein patch is planned
3. **Isolate** common, external, and internal carotid arteries
4. **Heparinize** with 100 mg/kg IV, then notify anesthesia and place atraumatic **clamps** on internal and common carotid arteries
5. Make longitudinal **arteriotomy**: open ICA anterolateral surface, from bulb to beyond border of atheromatous plaque
6. If shunting planned, first insert **shunt** proximally into common carotid, allow blood to flush air out of lumen, then insert distal end into internal carotid artery
7. Create **endarterectomy** dissection plane in mid to outer media, elevate circumferentially with spatula, beginning proximally and extending distally, allowing for feathering at distal extent; avoid creating flap (or secure with suture if occurs)
8. **Close** arteriotomy with a running 6-0 polypropylene suture, usually with prosthetic or vein patch (e.g., saphenous or double-layer facial vein)
9. Just prior to completing suture line, **release** clamps in the following order to de-air and direct any debris into ECA rather than ICA: external, common, then internal carotid artery; reinforce suture line if needed to achieve hemostasis
10. Consider closed suction drain; **close** platysma and skin

Postop: Monitor cardiac and neuro status closely, avoid hypertension; carotid thrombosis warrants emergent re-exploration; if resp distress from hematoma, obtain airway control, open wound at bedside if necessary (and take emergently to OR)

Risks: MI, stroke/hyperperfusion syndrome, acute thrombosis, hemorrhage (± airway compromise), infection, restenosis, nerve injury (recurrent laryngeal [5–7%], potentially requiring trach. if contralat. nerve is also compromised; superior laryngeal [1–3%]; spinal accessory [0.5–1%]; hypoglossal [4–6%]; marginal mandibular [1–3%])

Femorofemoral Bypass

Indications:

Emergent — Acute occlusion of unilateral CIA and/or EIA from IABP
Elective — Disabling claudication, rest pain, gangrene or ulceration in the presence of high-grade ipsilateral stenosis/occlusion of CIA and/or EIA; occlusion of one limb of aortofemoral graft when thrombectomy not possible; following ligation of iliac artery or aortofemoral graft eroded by infection; also, in combination with axillofemoral grafting in management of high-grade bilateral iliac stenoses in *high-risk* patients; and in management of mycotic AAA where unsafe to place a prosthetic graft in situ

Setup: Anesthesia: local (emergent IABP occlusions in ICU), spinal, epidural or general;
Position = Supine, Foley; ECG, oximetry, ±A-line, PA catheter only for high-risk cardiac pts; careful cleansing and preparation of the groins prior to incision; prep skin from upper abdomen to feet but drape narrowly, leaving only lower abdomen, and bilateral groins visible

Procedure: (Consider two-team approach)

1. Bilateral vertical **incisions** overlying femoral pulses exposing inguinal ligaments superiorly, **ligate** lymphatics to prevent postoperative lymphocele
2. **Expose CFAs** bilaterally from inguinal ligaments to their bifurcations
3. If SFA occluded, **expose** enough **profunda** to allow endarterectomy
4. Select 6 or 8 mm PTFE or polyester **graft**, cut to appropriate size
5. **Tunnel** graft using a curved tunneling device approximating the diameter of the graft
6. Obtain proximal and distal **control** of CFA/SFA/PFA and administer **heparin** 100 U/kg
7. Perform **proximal anastomosis** side-to-end on healthiest portion of CFA/SFA/PFA; perform endarterectomy if necessary
8. Perform **distal anastomosis** to optimize runoff: e.g., cross PFA takeoff with end to side anastomosis if SFA occluded, and perform endarterectomy if necessary
9. **Assess** ankle/foot vascular status (with doppler if necessary), consider arteriogram
10. Ensure **hemostasis**, **close** in two layers

Risks/Results: Major acute in 5%: local hemorrhage, acute thrombosis, MI, stroke, GI hemorrhage, DVT/PE, wound infection/dehiscence, graft infection, operative mortality (2%); 5 yr primary patency 64%; 5 yr secondary patency 69%

Femoropopliteal Bypass

Indications:
Disabling claudication, rest pain, gangrene or ulceration in the presence of high-grade ipsilateral stenosis/occlusion of SFA

Setup: **Anesthesia**: epidural preferable, spinal or general. **Position**: Supine with ipsilateral thigh abducted, and flexed at hip and knee, Foley; ECG, oximetry, ±A-line, CVP linc, PA catheter for high-risk cardiac pts; careful cleansing and preparation of the groins prior to incision; prep skin from upper abdomen to feet bilaterally and circumferentially but drape narrowly, leaving only ipsilateral groin and medial thigh and leg visible

Procedure (Reversed SVG):
1. Ipsilateral vertical groin **incision** midway between pubic tubercle and ASIS, **ligate** lymphatics to prevent postoperative lymphocele or lymphorrhea
2. Expose saphenofemoral juction; divide **SV** at jn; dissect inferiorly, ligate/divide tributaries; make short-segment, non-continuous incisions overlying SV to obtain appropriate length, one incision should also serve as exposure for popliteal artery.
3. Cannulate proximal end of **SVG** and secure cannula in place; place atraumatic bulldog clamp on distal end; gently distend SVG with fluid; control leaks with fine suture; use fine sutures or marking pen to mark longitudinal orientation (store submerged)
4. **Expose CFA** from inguinal lig. to bifurcation; dissect out profunda if CFA diseased
5. Expose popliteal artery between sartorius and vastus medialis within adductor canal
6. Administer **heparin** 100 U/kg; clamp prox. and dist. on **CFA**; make longitudinal arteriotomy 2X longer than vessel diameter, T-incision in distal (smaller end of) SVG; side-to-end **anastomosis** with running 6-0 or 7-0 polypropylene sutures
7. Place **tunnel**ing device under sartorius in popliteal incision and bring out through femoral incision; attach to free end of SVG and pull back out through popliteal incision; orient the graft using marking sutures to ensure no twisting
8. Clamp prox. and dist. on **popliteal**; longitudinal arteriotomy, end-to-side **anastomosis**
9. Ensure **hemostasis**, assess ankle/foot vascular status; consider completion A-gram
10. **Close** incisions in two layers

F/U: ASA 81 or 325mg QD. Clinic 2 wks postop to √Sx, wound, pulses, ABI. Q3 months for ABI and duplex scanning; Q6 months thereafter

Risks: Local hemorrhage, acute thrombosis, MI, stroke, GI hemorrhage, DVT/PE, wound infection/dehiscence, graft infection, leg edema, saphenous neuropathy, pseudoaneurysm. 5 yr primary patency 70%; 5 yr secondary patency 80% (above-knee)

Femorotibial/Femorodistal Bypass

Indications:
Disabling claudication in exceptional cases, rest pn, gangrene or ulceration in the presence of high-grade ipsilateral occlusion of SFA, and popliteal arteries

Setup: **Anesthesia**: epidural preferable, spinal or general. **Position**: Supine with ipsilateral thigh abducted, and flexed at hip and knee, Foley; ECG, oximetry, ±A-line, CVP line, PA catheter for high-risk cardiac patients; careful cleansing of groin prior to procedure; prep skin from upper abdomen to feet bilaterally and circumferentially but drape narrowly, leaving only ipsilateral groin and medial thigh; leave leg visible over site of distal anastomosis

Procedure: (Procedure similar to femoropopliteal bypass, but must be individualized to best runoff vessel)

1. Harvest full length of ipsilateral **saphenous** vein as described (note: using transposed *non*reversed SVG allows better size-matching than RSVG, but valves must by lysed)
2. **Contralateral** vein may be used if ipsilateral vein not available; may also use **composite** grafts of bilateral lesser saphenous veins or cephalic veins as needed
3. **Exposure** of **posterior tibial** (PTA) and **peroneal** arteries best performed through a medial leg incision, just posterior to tibia; PTA is covered only by skin, fascia and connective tissue, and can be identified by developing a plane between the flexor digitorum longus anteriorly and the gastrocnemius/soleus group posteriorly; avoid injury to SV or tibial nerves.
4. **Peroneal artery** is just deep to the posterior tibial; expose by developing plane between flexor hallucis longis and tibialis posterior and dividing intermuscular septum.
5. **Anterior tibial artery** (ATA) best exposed through anterolateral vertical leg incision; opening the anterior compartment and dividing the intermuscular septum between the extensor hallucis longis and the tibialis anterior; identify ATA deep in the anterior compartment.
6. **Grafts** are best tunneled in an intramuscular position as in femoropopliteal bypassing
7. **Assess** ankle/foot vascular status (with doppler if necessary), selective completion arteriography for complicated or technically problematic procedures
8. **Close** incisions in two layers

Postop: ASA 81 or 325mg QD, consider addition of other platelet inhibitors or anticoagulant; Clinic 2 wks postop to √Sx, wound, pulses, ABI. Q3 months for ABI and duplex scanning; Q6 months thereafter

Risks: Local hemorrhage, acute thrombosis, MI, stroke, GI hemorrhage, DVT/PE, wound infection/dehiscence, graft infection, leg edema, saphenous neuropathy, pseudoaneurysm; patency rates lower than for femoropopliteal bypass

Hemodialysis Access: Intravenous Dialysis Catheter Placement

Indications:

1. Need for dialysis access and immediate use anticipated; often used after failed salvage of A-V fistula
2. Short term dialysis

Setup: Position = supine; place towel beneath shoulders, prep both sides of neck, chest

Procedure:

1. For **IJ approach** — With head turned to contralat. side, insert introducer needle at apex of triangle formed by two heads of the SCM; aim needle toward ipsilat. nipple at 45º angle, aspirate in gentle, short bursts while advancing needle until vein is entered
2. For **SC approach** — Align introducer needle with deltopectoral groove, insert needle 1–2 cm inferior to clavicle, target portion of vein = postage-stamp-sized area deep to clavicle at insertion of medial head of SCM; pass needle just beneath the clavicle, aspirate in short bursts while advancing needle until vein is entered
3. Advance **guidewire** through introducer, using fluoro. to confirm location in SVC, make stab incision adjacent to wire
4. Incise skin over anterior chest, 5–10 cm from puncture site; **tunnel** dialysis catheter subcutaneously from the anterior chest to wire exit site, such that cuff lies subcutaneously ~ 2 cm from the anterior chest incision (note: placing further from catheter exit site allows more room for re-positioning catheter if needed, but makes eventual removal of the catheter more difficult)
5. Determine the approximate **length** of catheter needed to place tip in SVC, then cut the excess catheter off at the distal end
6. **Dilate** over guidewire and advance break-away sheath with inner cannula over guidewire
7. **Remove** the inner cannula and guidewire together, leaving break-away sheath in place, while taking precautions to prevent air from entering sheath
8. Quickly **insert** catheter tip into lumen of the sheath, advance into SVC, and remove break-away sheath
9. Use fluoroscopy to **confirm** catheter tip near SVC/RA junction, flush catheter with heparinized saline, close incisions, secure catheter, check patency and flush again, fill catheter with concentrated heparin solution
10. Obtain postoperative **chest film** to document catheter position and identify complications (always check yourself)

Postop: CXR in recovery room to R/O pneumothorax, re-confirm position

Risks: Pneumo/hemothorax; major hemorrhage; minor bleeding from incisions (can be due to excessive heparin flush, usually resolved with manual pressure); infection (site, tunnel, or line sepsis), arrhythmia, cardiac rupture, nerve injury, air embolus, DVT/PE

Hemodialysis Access: Brescia/Cimino Fistula

Indications:

Current or imminent need for hemodialysis in patient with chronic ESRD

Setup: **Anesthesia** — local with IV sedation preferable; can use axillary block or general. **Position** — Supine with operative arm abducted and laid upon a table. Circumferential prep of arm from hand to shoulder

Procedure: (Side-to-side radiocephalic)

1. Make longitudinal **incision** over radial artery approximately 2 cm proximal to the wrist
2. **Mobilize** a length of **radial artery** and **cephalic vein** such that the two can be positioned side-to-side without tension; use careful no-touch dissection to avoid inducing spasm
3. Apply **vessel loops** around the artery and vein proximally and distally
4. **Clamp vein and artery** proximally and distally
5. Make longitudinal **arteriotomy and venotomy** (5–10 mm long)
6. Perform side-to-side **anastomosis** between artery and vein, consider ligating vein distally if flow through fistula is poor
7. Establish meticulous **hemostasis**
8. **Assess** radial pulse and perfusion in hand
9. **Close** in two layers
10. If urgent dialysis required, **intravenous dialysis catheter** may be placed during the same procedure

Postop Management: No circumferential bandages; no venipuncture or IV lines in operative arm; DDAVP 0.3μg/kg may ameliorate wound bleeding

Risks: Local hemorrhage, acute thrombosis, steal (should prompt urgent ligation or revision), aggravation of CHF, failure to mature

Follow-up: Maturation of fistula should be assessed at 4–6 weeks

Hemodialysis Access: Basilic Vein Transposition AV Graft — Upper Arm [37]

Indications:

Permanent access for hemodialysis; second choice procedure if failed primary wrist fistula (AVF), or patients lacking adequate veins for a primary wrist AVF

Setup:

Position = supine; ECG, oximetry
Prep includes entire hand from the tips of the fingers to the axilla as well as ipsilateral shoulder and chest wall

Procedure:

1. Make longitudinal **incision** over medial aspect of the distal upper arm overlying brachial pulse ~ 2 cm proximal to elbow crease
2. Identify **basilic vein**, extend proximally to level of axilla following the course of basilic vein
3. Leave an intact skin bridge at the elbow crease, and dissect out the **distal segment** of basilic vein, ligating side branches as needed
4. **Ligate and transect** the distal basilic vein (2-0 or 3-0 silk)
5. **Clamp** the basilic vein **proximally**, and flush graft with heparinized saline
6. Dissect out the **brachial artery** and clamp proximally and distally
7. **Tunnel** the basilic vein graft subcutaneously with tunneling device or long, curved clamp to the region of brachial artery
8. Construct end-to-side basilic vein to brachial artery **anastomosis** with running 6-0 polypropylene
9. Irrigate, ensure hemostasis, and **close** wounds in layers with 3-0 ± 4-0 absorbable sutures
10. **Check** arm pulses, graft for bruit, thrill

Risks: Major acute 1–5%: local hemorrhage, thrombosis, steal syndrome <1%

Follow-up: Graft allowed to mature for at least 8 weeks prior to using

Hemodialysis Access: PTFE AV Graft — Upper Extremity

Indications:

Current or imminent need for hemodialysis in patient with chronic ESRD and inadequate venous anatomy for primary fistula; failed prior dialysis access with poor venous anatomy

Setup: **Anesthesia** — local with IV sedation preferable; can use axillary block or general. **Position** — supine with operative arm abducted and laid on a table. Circumferential prep of arm from hand to shoulder and base of neck

Procedure:

1. **Select** artery (> 4 mm diam.) with unobstructed flow for inflow, as distal as possible to allow for subsequent access procedures and any 4 mm or larger vein with unobstructed outflow; common combinations include the radial artery and median cubital vein below elbow; distal brachial artery and median cubital vein above elbow; distal brachial artery and distal basilic vein (near axilla)
2. Make longitudinal **incision** over the respective artery and vein
3. **Dissect** out a length of artery and vein, obtaining proximal and distal **control** of each
4. Cut appropriate length of 6 mm PTFE **graft** and **tunnel** it between the sites planned for arterial and venous anastomosis; counter incision may be needed for loop grafts
5. **Clamp vein** proximally and distally
6. Perform angled end-to-side **anastomosis** between graft and **vein**; avoid extraneous puncture holes on graft
7. Clamp and perform end-to-side **anastomosis** between graft and **artery**
8. Ensure **hemostasis**
9. Assess radial **pulse**, check for **thrill** in graft (and augmentation with distal occlusion)
10. **Close** in two layers

Postop: No circumferential bandages; no venipuncture or IV lines in operative arm; DDAVP 0.3µg/kg may ameliorate wound bleeding if problematic

Risks: Local hemorrhage, acute thrombosis, steal (requires urgent graft revision to improve hand perfusion), infection, aggravation of CHF

Portasystemic Shunt: Interposition Mesocaval Shunt

Indications:

Emergent — Uncontrolled variceal hemorrhage;
Elective — Recurrent esophageal variceal hemorrhage, with Child's A or B Cirrhosis or Budd Chiari Syndrome

Setup: **Anesthesia**: general; **Position**: Supine, Foley; ECG, oximetry, A-line, PA catheter. Prep skin from clavicles to groins bilaterally but drape narrowly, leaving only region of planned incision exposed

Procedure:

1. Long upper midline or bilateral subcostal **incision**, avoid injury to umbilical varices
2. **Explore** abd and liver for hepatoma; consider performing liver biopsy if indicated
3. **Reflect** greater omentum and transverse mesocolon cephalad
4. Make generous transverse incision at base of transverse mesocolon and expose **SMV** usually near midline
5. Carefully **ligate** adjacent engorged **lymphatic** channels
6. **Mobilize** 6-7cm segment of **SMV** caudally from inferior margin of pancreas; divide branches from uncinate process and double loop posterior mesenteric branch with vessel loop
7. Opening right colon mesentery, mobilize 2nd and 3rd portions of duodenum and clean 6-7 cm length of **IVC** anteriorly and laterally and divide tissue of right colon mesentery between IVC and SMV
8. Controlling the **IVC** with side-biting clamp, perform end-to-side **anastomosis** of polyester **graft** tailored to size of IVC and SMV (typically 8 or 10 mm diameter)
9. Obtain proximal and distal control on SMV with clamps, cut graft to length, **anastomose SMV** to **graft**, side-to-end, vent graft as clamps are removed; take shunted and unshunted pressure measurements
10. **Close abdomen** in standard fashion; consider retention sutures

Postop: ICU; colloid fluids; careful fluid management to maximize organ perfusion while minimizing ascites; NGT, GI prophylaxis; start spironolactone on POD 3; careful F/U and management of ascites, encephalopathy, liver disease, aggressive ethanol cessation intervention as appropriate

Risks: Rebleeding, shunt occlusion, encephalopathy, ascites (diuretics), chylous ascites (Rx: bowel rest, TPN, repeated paracentesis)

Portasystemic Shunt: Distal Splenorenal Shunt

Indications:

***Emergent*:** Uncontrolled variceal hemorrhage;
***Elective*:** Recurrent esophageal variceal hemorrhage, with Child's A or B cirrhosis or portal vein thrombosis; bleeding gastric varices

Setup: **Anesthesia**: general. **Position**: Supine, Foley; ECG, oximetry, A-line, ±PA catheter; prep skin from clavicles to groins bilaterally but drape narrowly, leaving only region of planned incision exposed

Procedure:

1. Long upper midline or extended left subcostal **incision**, avoid umbilical varices; **explore** abdomen, perform liver biopsy if indicated
2. **Divide** all extra-anatomic vascular attachments to the spleen to avoid inadvertent capsular injury
3. Enter lesser sac through gastrocolic omentum, **dividing** the right gastroepiploic vein but leaving the artery intact; preserve short gastric and left gastroepiploic arteries
4. Enter retroperitoneum along the inferior border of body and tail of pancreas, carefully ligate large **lymphatic** channels and mobilize pancreas superomedially
5. **Ligate IMV** where it joins splenic vein
6. Carefully **mobilize** the **splenic vein** for 6–7 cm from proximally from its junction with the SMV beginning posteriorly, and then carefully ligating and dividing the tributaries emanating from the pancreas along its anterior surface; ligate and divide the coronary vein where it meets the portal vein
7. **Expose left renal vein** by reflecting the transverse colon and dividing the ligament of Treitz, and dissecting it free of surrounding attachments; ligate and divide left adrenal vein
8. If patient has normal coagulation, administer **heparin** 100 U/kg; using two vascular clamps, **divide** the **splenic vein** at its junction with the SMV, and oversew it so that there is no blind pouch; release cephalad retraction of pancreas to ensure that there is an adequate length of splenic vein.
9. Place a side-biting clamp on left renal vein and **anastomose** splenic vein to left renal vein end-to-side with 5-0 polypropylene
10. **Close** abdomen in standard fashion; consider retention sutures

Postop: ICU; colloid fluids; careful fluid management to maximize organ perfusion while minimizing ascites; NGT, GI prophylaxis, 24 hrs of IV 2nd generation cephalosporins; start spironolactone on POD 3; careful F/U and management of ascites, encephalopathy, liver disease, aggressive ethanol cessation intervention

Risks: Rebleeding in 5–7%; shunt occlusion in 5%; encephalopathy: 5% early; 10–15% at 3 years; ascites (diuretics); chylous ascites (Rx: bowel rest, TPN, repeated paracentesis)

Section 3
PEDIATRIC SURGERY

Congenital Diaphragmatic Hernia — Repair

Indications:

***Emergent*:** Medical, not surgical, emergency due to pulmonary hypoplasia and inadequate ventilation/oxygenation; mainstays of treatment are cautious ventilatory management, possibly alkalinization, may require high frequency jet ventilation or ECMO
***Elective*:** Repair once baby stabilized medically

Special cases: Consider other anomalies (15–25%, most commonly cardiovascular); intestinal malrotation is universally present

Setup: Orogastric tube at birth to decompress stomach/aspirate swallowed air. Position = supine

Procedure:

1. Typically a transabdominal approach through a **left subcostal** incision
2. **Reduce** viscera from the chest (may require enlarging the defect)
3. **Dissect** out posterior leaflet of diaphragm from peritoneum and pleura
4. **Excise** hernia **sac** if present
5. Mattress 2-0 non-absorbable sutures to **close** diaphragmatic defect; may need to include rib(s) if no posterior rim (especially the lateral margin)
6. **May** use synthetic material or muscle **flaps** for large defect
7. If a chest tube is placed, it should be connected to **underwater seal** only to prevent excessive mediastinal shift when suction is applied
8. **Consider** correcting malrotation and lysing Ladd's bands
9. **Close** by stretching abdominal wall to facilitate fascial closure
10. It is occasionally necessary to create a **ventral hernia** to avoid excessive increases in intra-abdominal pressure, which adversely affect compliance and gas exchange

Risks: Post-op ventilatory failure, pneumothorax from barotrauma (pre or post-op), disruption of repair with recurrence, postop hemorrhage, particularly if temporally associated with ECMO, midgut volvulus

Foreign Body: Esophageal

Indications: Presence of esophageal foreign body; all esophageal foreign bodies should be removed once discovered (urgent), particularly if the patient is unable to handle secretions

Studies: PA and lateral chest films that include neck and abdomen; barium swallow is rarely necessary unless the object is not radiopaque

Special cases:

1. Neglected foreign bodies may present as aspiration pneumonia, fever, cough, or symptoms of esophageal perforation
2. Remove all batteries and other objects likely to cause corrosion or perforation

Setup: Position = supine

Procedure:

Non-operative — drinking **warm, carbonated beverage** may force object into stomach, serial films required to follow progress through GI tract
Operative

1. **Fluoroscopy** — place Foley beyond object under fluoroscopic guidance; inflate balloon with radio-opaque solution and withdraw catheter
2. Rigid **Esophagoscopy**
    a) Open mouth, protect teeth, **introduce esophagoscope** over base of tongue into esophagus under direct vision
    b) **Retrieve** object with forceps or balloon catheter and retrieve by withdrawing the entire apparatus

Risks: Esophageal perforation or laceration

F/U: If object manipulated into stomach and cannot be retrieved, serial abdominal films over several weeks to follow progression out of GI tract may be required

Foreign Body Aspiration

Indications: History of choking in a child of appropriate age; sudden onset of respiratory symptoms, usually unilateral; radiographic confirmation of foreign body

Note: Sudden coughing, choking, voice loss, dyspnea, stridor, retractions, wheezing; attempt to determine nature of foreign body and time elapsed

Studies: Expiration films and/or fluoroscopy may show hyperaeration on affected side due to air trapping

Procedures:

Non-operative

1. Turn child upside down with **back blows**
2. **Consider Heimlich** maneuver only for witnessed choking episode

Operative

1. **Direct laryngoscopy** with removal of object if in pharynx or larynx (a McGill forceps will usually suffice)
2. **Bronchoscopy** — rigid more versatile
   a. Visualize **vocal cords** with laryngoscope
   b. **Introduce** rigid bronchoscope through cords
   c. **Remove** foreign body with grasping forces or balloon catheter
3. **Treat** postobstructive pneumonia, if present; persistent reactive airway symptoms may require treatment with bronchodilators or steroids

Risks: Continued partial airway obstruction from edema, secretions, blood, or mucus; perforation of trachea, pneumomediastinum, pneumothorax, hypoxic injury

Gastroschisis

Indications: Diagnosis by prenatal ultrasound or newborn examination

Note:

1. Most found on prenatal U/S; results may be improved by early delivery if there is ultrasound evidence of bowel wall thickening/inflammation, assuming satisfactory maturity
2. Typically 2–4 cm diameter defect lateral to normal umbilical cord; no peritoneal covering
3. Almost always to right of umbilical cord

Setup: Position = supine with orogastric tube

Procedure: Options include primary closure, skin closure with secondary hernia repair, and Silastic silo with gradual closure; primary closure usually possible

1. Consider vertical **extension** of defect to facilitate reduction of herniated viscera
2. **Inspect** abdominal contents, especially for associated intestinal atresia
3. **Milk** meconium and air from the bowel to reduce volume
4. Manually **stretch** abdominal wall
5. **Replace** viscera into abdomen
6. **Monitor** ventilation pressures; intragastric and intravesical pressures may also be indicative of excessive intra-abdominal pressure
7. **Close** fascia primarily, if possible; otherwise, attach a Silastic sheet to the edge of the fascial defect to create the silo for gradual reduction
8. Consider central line for **TPN**

Risks: Respiratory insufficiency and poor venous return due to excessive intra-abdominal pressure post reduction, ischemia of flaps, hemorrhage, cellulitis, fasciitis, abdominal wall hernia, inguinal hernias. Anticipate excessive loss of protein-rich peritoneal fluid from a silo closure, which must be replaced to minimize bowel edema and facilitate reduction

Low Imperforate Anus: Cutback Anoplasty, Transposition Anoplasty or Limited Posterior Sagittal Anoplasty

Indications: Diagnosis on newborn physical examination; occasionally presents later due to constipation or problems with defecation

Notes: Majority of low lesions (2/3) occur in females; abnormal position of the anal orifice on the perineum or vagina, failure to pass meconium

Studies: Evaluate associated anomalies including cardiac (examination, echocardiogram), axial spine (radiograph), limbs (examination, radiograph), tracheoesophageal anomalies, urinary system (ultrasound, possibly voiding cystourethrogram) and tethered cord (ultrasound, possibly MRI.) Ultrasound and/or contrast studies may help localize the level of the rectal pouch.

Setup: Position = prone jackknife

Procedure (transposition or limited posterior sagital anoplasty):

1. **Identify** the center of the sphincteric complex with nerve stimulator and mark with indelible marker
2. **Circumferential incision** around the opening of the fistula; it is very important to preserve the mucosa of the fistula tract
3. Using the nerve stimulator, the muscles of the sphincteric complex are divided in layers and tagged **exactly in the midline**
4. **Dissect** rectal pouch sufficiently to create the neoanus without tension
5. **Reconstruct** external sphincter around the neoanus in layers and complete the mucosa to skin anastomosis; calibrate the neoanus with dilators

Risks: Hemorrhage, sepsis, wound complications, anal stenosis; incontinence or problems with defecation should be uncommon with low lesions

High Imperforate Anus: Posterior Sagital Anorectoplasty [42]

Indications: Diagnosis on newborn physical examination; occasionally presents with evidence of distal intestinal obstruction

Notes: The majority of high lesions are found in males (2/3) and are usually associated with fistulas to the urinary tract; high lesions in females often have associated fistulas to the upper vagina, and may be associated with uterine anomalies such as uterus didelphus. Urinary fistulas are confirmed by the presence of air or meconium in the urine.

Studies:

1. Invertogram - baby upside down after enough time has passed to allow air to reach distal GI tract, often will show level of rectum and gas in bladder; high imperforate anus will show rectal stump above pubo-coccygeal line; retained meconium in the rectal pouch can be misleading
2. Ultrasound examination will accurately demonstrate the position of the blind rectal pouch relative to the pelvic floor
3. Evaluate associated anomalies including cardiac (examination, echocardiogram), axial spine (radiograph), limbs (examination, radiograph), tracheoesophageal anomalies and tethered cord (ultrasound, possibly MRI.)
4. Retrograde urethragram to visualize the fistula and rectal pouch, as indicated

Setup: Position = prone jackknife

Procedure:

1. **High** lesions are usually best managed by diverting **colostomy** in the newborn, followed by **posterior sagital anorectoplasty** at 6–12 months of age
2. Locate the center of the **sphincteric complex** using the nerve stimulator and mark with indelible ink
3. **Divide perineal musculature** precisely in midline using the nerve stimulator, marking each layer with sutures
4. Divide and oversew the **fistula**
5. **Mobilize** rectal pouch to reach the perineum without tension
6. **Reconstruct** muscles of the pelvic floor around newly pulled through rectum
7. **Complete** construction of the **neoanus** with interrupted sutures and calibrate

Risks: Sepsis, wound complications, anal stenosis, anal mucosal prolapse, incontinence

Pediatric Inguinal Hernia Repair

Indications:

Emergent – Strangulation, incarceration
Urgent – Incarceration with difficult reduction, repair same admission
Elective – Presence of hernia; in hospitalized premature infants, repair prior to d/c home

Setup: Position = supine

Procedure: (Males)

1. Make transverse skin **incision** in groin skin crease, incise Scarpa's, bluntly dissect tissue overlying external oblique
2. Identify external inguinal ring, then incise **external oblique**, avoiding injury to ilioinguinal nerve
3. **Mobilize** the spermatic **cord**
4. **Identify** hernia **sac** anterior and medial to cord
5. **Dissect sac away** from cord structures, avoiding injury to vas deferens, vessels
6. **Divide** empty **sac** between hemostats
7. Twist sac 1–2 turns and **ligate sac** at level of internal ring
8. May remove **distal sac** or open and leave in situ
9. **Close** wound in layers
10. **Consider** contralateral exploration in patients with suggestive physical findings or at increased risk of bilaterality (prematurity, abdominal wall defect, CDH, hydrocephalus with V-P shunt, etc.)

Risks: Hemorrhage, infection, testicular atrophy, injury to vas deferens, spermatic vessels; postanesthetic apnea in premature infant with conceptual age less than 60 weeks

Intussusception

Indications:

Emergent – Shock, peritonitis
Urgent – Failed barium/air reduction

Note: Typically infant, 5-10 months, male predominance; otherwise healthy child with sudden onset of colicky pain often manifested by retraction of legs to abdomen; attacks usually 5-20 minutes apart, child often exhausted between bouts. Emesis and current jelly stools are late findings; on exam, sausage shaped mass may be palpated, rectal exam may reveal tip of intussusception +/– blood.

Studies:

1. Supine/upright radiograph may be normal to partial/complete intestinal obstruction
2. U/S in some centers with "target" or "pseudokidney"
3. Barium or air enema diagnostic and therapeutic in up to 75% of cases; the intussusception must be reduced completely with free reflux of contrast into the terminal ileum

Setup: Position = Supine with orogastric or nasogastric tube

Procedure:

1. Make transverse infra-umbilical or RLQ **incision**
2. **Deliver** intussusception into wound
3. Gentle **pressure** applied to entire mass to decrease edema
4. Gentle and continuous **massage** from distal to proximal (much like squeezing a tube of toothpaste)
5. **Never** pull ends apart
6. **Resect** with end-to-end anastomosis **if** manual **reduction fails**, reduced bowel is **gangrenous**, or specific **lead point** identified (Meckel's, polyp, etc)
7. **Consider** appendectomy
8. **Close**

Risks: Hemorrhage, necrosis of unresected compromised bowel, recurrence, wound infection, ileus

Ladd's Procedure: Malrotation with Mid-gut Volvulus

Indications:

Emergent – Bilious vomiting in children in malrotation with mid-gut volvulus and is a surgical emergency until proven otherwise due to the catastrophic nature of the problem
Elective – Incidental finding of malrotation on UGI obtained for other reasons

Studies:

1. Plain film of abdomen showing gasless abdomen or consistent with obstruction; however, the plain radiograph may be completely normal, and a normal examination does not exclude the diagnosis
2. UGI if peritonitis absent and child stable
3. Consider barium enema

Setup: Position = Supine; OG tube

Procedure:

1. Optimal approach is via **supra-umbilical transverse** incision
2. **Deliver** intestines into wound
3. Rotate bowel **counterclockwise** to correct the volvulus
4. **Fan** out small bowel over abdominal wall, spread out mesentery as much as possible
5. Incise **Ladd's bands** across the duodenum; the mobilized duodenum should lie along the right side of the spine.
6. Continue dissection of bands until **cecum**/ascending colon lies in LUQ, **small bowel** on right side of abdomen
7. Perform **appendectomy**
8. Assess bowel for **viability; if the intestine is necrotic, resect** as little as possible – consider a second-look procedure if in doubt
9. **Close** abdomen

Risks: Wound infection, bleeding, sepsis, unresected compromised or necrotic bowel

Necrotizing Enterocolitis — Surgical Management

Indications:

Emergent – Pneumoperitoneum, clinical deterioration, abdominal wall erythema, abdominal mass, fixed bowel loop; the majority of patients are premature, the incidence increasing with the degree of immaturity

Studies:

Generally, the patient should be taken to the operating room shortly after diagnosis. Stabilization should include volume resuscitation, correction of acidosis and correction of coagulopathy, if present. This may be facilitated by drainage of the peritoneal cavity via a penrose drain placed under local anesthesia, with full exploration deferred several hours.

Procedure:

1. Right **transverse supra-umbilical** incision
2. Send **peritoneal fluid** for gram stain, C&S
3. **Inspect** entire GI tract for perforation/necrosis
4. **Resect** perforated/necrotic bowel
5. **Preserve** as much length of intestine as possible; exteriorize the ends
6. Multiple **ostomies** may be required to preserve length where involvement is segmental
7. Multiple **re-explorations** to assess viability may be required
8. If needed, place **central line** for TPN

Risks: Death, wound complications, intestinal strictures (warrants contrast study of distal bowel to r/o stricture prior to stoma closure), hemorrhage

Nissen Fundoplication

Indications:

GER complicated by aspiration (apnea, recurrent infections, lung abscess, reactive airways disease), stricture, or persistent vomiting with failure to thrive, or GER refractory to medical therapy

Studies: May include some combination of the following:

1. Barium swallow/ UGI
2. 24 hr esophageal pH monitoring
3. Radionuclide gastric emptying study (an associated emptying procedure may be indicated)
4. Esophagoscopy with biopsy

Setup: Position = supine

Procedure:

1. Midline **incision**
2. Mobilize the lateral segment of the left lobe of the liver and retract to the right, **exposing** the **esophageal hiatus**
3. Divide peritoneum over esophagus and **mobilize**
4. **Close crura** (optional)
5. Divide **short gastrics** if needed to adequately mobilize fundus
6. **Wrap** greater curvature of fundus behind intra-abdominal esophagus
7. **Suture** to self and anterior esophagus over dilator to create a circumferential wrap of fundus around the distal esophagus
8. Construct **2–3 cm long** wrap
9. **Consider Stamm gastrostomy** (often used in children with CNS dysfunction and poor feeding — procedure the same as in adult)
10. **Consider pyloroplasty** with poor gastric emptying (same as in adult)

Risks: Inability to vomit or burp, gas bloat syndrome, esophageal obstruction, vagal nerve injury resulting in delayed gastric emptying, post-op intestinal obstruction; persistent gagging and retching is relatively common, particularly in neurologically impaired patients

Omphalocele Closure

Indications:

Prenatal diagnosis by ultrasound or newborn physical examination

Note: Intestines covered by sac with umbilical cord arising out of sac

Studies: Due to high incidence of other anomalies, may require renal or cardiac U/S, chromosomal analysis; also associated with other midline defects (Pentalogy of Cantrell). Rarely associated with Beckwith-Wiedeman syndrome (macroglossia, islet cell hyperplasia) which can cause clinically significant hypoglycemia.

Setup: Position = Supine; orogastric tube

Procedures:

Primary closure

1. **Excise** omphalocele **sac**, inspect abdomen, milk intestinal contents proximally and distally to decrease volume
2. Manually **stretch** abdominal cavity
3. **Close** fascia primarily if possible, continuously monitoring ventilation pressures (intragastric and intravesicle pressures may also be of value)

Sialastic Silo

1. **Suture silastic** sheet to border of fascial defect; consider enlarging the defect to present ischemia of the herniated viscera and facilitate reduction
2. **Gradually reduce** silo contents into abdomen (2–4 days)
3. **Remove silo** and **close** fascia in operating room
4. **Consider** central line for TPN

Risks: Respiratory insufficiency, inadequate renal perfusion and/or poor venous return to heart if closure too tight, ischemia of skin/muscle flaps, cellulitis, fasciitis, hemorrhage

Pyloromyotomy

Indications:

Pyloric stenosis (after correction of fluid deficits, electrolyte abnormalities)

Note: 2–6 week old previously healthy baby with recent onset of projectile, non-bilious vomiting. Vomiting usually 30–60 min post feeding, may have visible gastric wave post feeding, palpable mass ("olive") just above and to right of umbilicus, firm, mobile. It is very important to correct existing fluid and electrolyte abnormalities preoperatively (typically a hypokalemic, hypochloremic metabolic alkalosis).

Studies: Consider U/S (or possibly barium UGI) if the "olive" is not palpable

Setup: Position = supine

Procedures:

1. **Transverse RUQ incision** over rectus
2. Deliver **pylorus** into wound
3. Carefully **incise serosa** over anterior/superior surface
4. Extend incision **proximally** onto gastric antrum
5. Extend incision **distally**, stopping approx 4 mm short of the palpable distal end of pylorus muscle
6. **Split** muscle with pylorus spreader or blunt end of scalpel until mucosal layer bulges thru
7. **Palpate** pylorus to assure both sides move independently of each other
8. Compress stomach to watch for bulging mucosa and to **R/O leak**
9. **Close** abdominal wound in layers

Risks: Perforation, wound infection, incomplete pyloromyotomy; persistent, less severe vomiting is somewhat common

Esophageal Atresia with Tracheoesophageal Fistula — Repair

Indications: Often suspected preoperatively due to polyhydramnios

Urgent – With fistula, once patient is stabilized, associated anomalies are evaluated and any pneumonitis has resolved

Elective – Pure atresia without fistula, 6–8 wks post gastrostomy tube placement

Studies:

1. Chest radiograph with frontal/lateral views w/ OG in place to localize the proximal esophageal pouch
2. Consider barium study to r/o proximal fistula
3. Pre-op cardiac echo to r/o anomaly (VACTERL) and determine the location of the aortic arch
4. Renal U/S to r/o renal agenesis
5. Consider intra-op bronchoscopy to r/o proximal fistula

Setup: Position = Left lateral decubitus

Procedure:

1. Right posterolateral extra-pleural **thoracotomy** (unless right-sided aortic arch in which case a left thoracotomy is used), enter chest via **4th** intercostal space
2. Extrapleural **dissection** posterior to azygous vein, **divide** and ligate azygous vein
3. **Divide fistula,** close tracheal side of fistula with interrupted non-absorbable sutures
4. **Dissect** proximal esophagus to thoracic inlet (look for proximal fistula), perform minimal distal esophageal dissection
5. **Consider** proximal **esophagomyotomy** to increase length
6. Construct single-layer **anastomosis**
7. Insert 8 or 10 Fr **OG tube**
8. Place extrapleural **chest tube**
9. Measure distance to anastomosis with suction catheter and **mark** catheter for use during suctioning so that anastomosis is not inadvertently disrupted
10. **Consider** a **gastrostomy** to minimize the risk of aspiration if the patient is not a satisfactory candidate for primary repair (prematurity, associated anomalies, clinically significant aspiration); however, the gastrostomy may result in a significant loss of tidal volume through the distal fistula, making the patient difficult or impossible to ventilate

Risks: Hemorrhage, tracheal injury, missed proximal fistula, anastomotic leak, infection, stricture, recurrent fistula, GE reflux, focal tracheomalacia; if the patient requires intubation postoperatively, it must be done carefully to avoid esophageal intubation and possible anastomotic disruption

Thyroglossal Duct Remnant Excision

Indications: Presence; may resect prior to or following resolution of infection

Note: Midline mass at or below hyoid. Mass is smooth, soft, nontender unless infected; the mass moves with protrusion of the tongue.

Studies: Consider thyroid scan if thyroid gland is not palpable (remnant may represent the **only** functional thyroid tissue)

Setup: Position = supine, neck extended (similar to positioning for thyroidectomy)

Procedure:

1. Make transverse skin **incision** in skin crease
2. **Dissect** cephalad to hyoid bone
3. **Excise** central portion of **hyoid** (Sistrunk procedure)
4. **Ligate base** of tract at floor of mouth with absorbable suture
5. **Close** wound in appropriate layers

Risks: Recurrence, wound infection

Section 4
OTHER INVASIVE PROCEDURES

Diagnostic Peritoneal Lavage — Open (*Closed in Italics*) [28,33,38]

Indications:

Blunt trauma: ? of intraabdominal injury, especially in hemodynamically unstable patient; inability to adequately or accurately assess abdomen, e.g. due to altered sensorium, spinal cord injury, injury to adjacent structures, or prolonged loss of contact with patient (surgery, studies, etc.); equivocal CT scan

Penetrating trauma (knife or low-velocity GSW) with questionable penetration of fascia

Contraindications:

Absolute: Indication for laparotomy

Relative: Cirrhosis, coagulopathy, pregnancy, morbid obesity, multiple prior abdominal surgeries (open technique in pregnancy or when adhesions anticipated)

Setup: Position = supine; OGT/NGT, Foley catheter in place, prep/drapes

Procedure:

1. **Infiltrate** skin with 1% lidocaine with epinephrine
2. Short midline infraumbilical skin **incision** 1/3 distance from umbilicus to pubic symphysis (*supra*umbilical in case of pelvic fx or pregnancy); *for closed technique, make stab incision*
3. **Dissect** down to linea alba with careful hemostasis (*omit in closed technique*)
4. 1–2 cm vertical incision in **fascia**, grasp edges with clamps and elevate; *omit for closed*
5. Introduce dialysis **catheter** (no stilette) blindly into peritoneal cavity toward pelvis (semi-open), or incise peritoneum and place catheter under direct vision (open) (*closed: advance needle toward pelvis while aspirating, thread guidewire, remove needle, then place catheter over wire and remove wire [Seldinger technique]*)
6. **Aspirate** peritoneal fluid with syringe (gross blood [$\geq$ 10 ml] or enteric contents = + tap)
7. If negative tap, **instill** one liter (10 ml/kg in children) warm LR or NS; distribute into all 4 quadrants, wait 5 minutes if feasible
8. Drop IV bag to floor and collect **effluent**
9. Remove catheter, **close** fascia and skin
10. Send lavage fluid for cell count/microscopic **analysis**

Interpretation:

Positive lavage result if lavage fluid appears in chest tube or foley, or has obvious bile or GI contents; or > 100,000 RBC/mm^3 (blunt trauma) [cutoff typically set lower (e.g., 10,000) in penetrating] or > 500 WBC/mm^3 in lavage fluid, or bacteria on gram stain of lavage fluid

Risks: Hemorrhage, injury to abdominal organs (e.g., bowel, bladder), peritonitis, wound infection

Endotracheal intubation — Rapid sequence

Indications: Unsuccessful bag-mask ventilation, airway protection in an unresponsive patient, respiratory insufficiency, cardiopulmonary arrest

Setup: Assure the presence of an oxygen source, bag and mask, intravenous access, fluid, medication for sedation, suction, laryngoscope, and several sizes of endotracheal tubes with stilettes

Procedure:

1. Place the patient **supine**, head tilted back
2. Apply **cricoid pressure**
3. **Hyperventilate** with 100% oxygen using bag and mask
4. Provide **analgesia and sedation**
5. Place the **laryngoscope** into the patient's mouth, displacing the tongue to the left, and advance the blade in the midline to the base of the tongue
6. **Visualize** the vocal **cords** and glottic opening and place the ET tube through the epiglottic opening, advancing the cuff 2 cm past the vocal cords into the trachea
7. **Inflate cuff** and **secure** tube with tape
8. **Auscultate** breath sounds bilaterally, check **end-tidal CO_2** when available
9. Obtain **CXR** to assess tube position
10. **If** intubation is **unsuccessful** for 30 seconds (or oxygen saturation falls below 90%), **ventilate** the patient with 100% oxygen before attempting again. If unable to bag/mask adequately and intubation is difficult, immediately perform cricothyroidotomy.

Risks: Injury to gums, teeth, or tongue; inappropriate placement of tube into esophagus (with possibility of perforation)

Tube Thoracostomy — Emergent [39]

Indications:

1. Evacuation of air (pneumothorax)
2. Evacuation of fluid (hemothorax, chylothorax, empyema, large pleural effusion)
3. Following needle decompression for presumed or actual tension pneumothorax

Setup:

1. Assure patent airway and adequate respirations (intubate patient if needed), administer oxygen, monitor pulse oximetry
2. Position patient supine with ipsilateral arm above head if possible
3. Choose entrance location at fifth interspace (nipple line) mid- to anterior axillary line
4. Have assistant set up and check function of pleural drainage device

Procedure:

1. Following rapid iodine prep and drape, infiltrate with lidocaine if pt awake, make 2–3 cm **transverse incision** through dermis; if patient is *un*stable the incision can be made directly over entrance interspace; if *stable*, incision is made one interspace below intended thoracostomy tube entrance location
2. **Dissect** through subcutaneous adipose tissue and muscle with Kelly clamp or scissors to create a cephalad-directed tunnel to fifth interspace
3. **Identify** superior edge of the 6th rib and seat tonsil or Kelly clamp in intercostal muscles of the 5th interspace
4. Stabilize closed clamp with *both hands* (nondominant one seated against chest to control depth), and carefully **penetrate** into pleural cavity
5. **Enlarge** thoracostomy by spreading the clamp and insert finger to confirm location in pleural cavity and that lung is not adhered to pleura
6. **Insert** 28-36 French chest tube (smaller for air only, larger for significant fluid) in a postero-cephalad direction to the apex of the chest cavity
7. **Attach** pleural drainage device
8. **Monitor** patient status and vital signs for immediate response, complications
9. **Secure** tube at incision with two "0" sutures and an umbilical tape
10. Obtain and view portable **chest film** for position of tube and residual pneumothorax or hemothorax

Risks: Hemorrhage; injury to lung parenchyma, heart, or intra-abdominal organ(s); inadequate drainage; infection (site infection or empyema)

Chapter IV

DATA ORGANIZATION, ORDERS, NOTES, DICTATIONS

Postop/Trauma Patient Summary Sheet:

Patient Name:		**Age, Sex:**
Hx #:	**Rm:**	**Attending:**

Procedure/Injury Mechanism:		Labs:
Injuries/Problems:		
#1:		
#2:		
#3:		
#4:		
#5:		
#6:		
#7:		
#8:		
#9:		
VS:		
Total fluids:		Studies:
Blood Products:		
Vent? Y / N Settings:		
Exam:		

Checklist (Check if completed, cross out or delete if irrelevant):			
☐ IV access ?	☐ Antibiotics ?	☐ Contrast for CT ?	☐ Films ordered ?
☐ NG in place ?	☐ Wound marker ?	☐ Chest tube (R / L)	☐ Consults* ?
☐ Foley in place ?	☐ OR called ?	☐ Tetanus toxoid ?	☐
*Consults — #1:		#2:	#3:
#4:	#5:	#6:	#7:

Asssessment:	**Plan:**

Orders (Composite)

Admission/Transfer/Postop Orders

- Admit/Transfer to (service, ward, attending)
- Diagnosis
- Condition
- Allergies
- Diet
- Activity
- VS (frequency)
- I/O (frequency)
- A-line/ECG/Central venous catheter monitoring
- SaO_2 monitoring q (frequency) or continuous
- Glucose checks q (frequency)
- Oxygen/Ventilator settings
- NG/OG to (low wall suction [LWS], gravity, etc)
- Drain(s) to (bulb suction or etc); recharge/empty/record q (frequency)
- Foley to gravity
- Chest tube to (water seal, -20 cm, or etc)
- Sequential compression devices while in bed
- Other nursing care (wound care, neuro checks, etc)
- IV fluids: type/rate
- Medications (representative):
    - Analgesics
    - Antibiotics
    - Anticoagulants (e.g., ASA, heparin, coumadin)
    - Drips
        - Anti-hypertensives
        - Anti-coagulants
        - Anti-arrhythmics
        - Insulin
    - β-blocker
    - Nitroglycerin patch/ointment
    - DVT prophylaxis
    - Gastric acid prophylaxis
    - Insulin/Oral hypoglycemic
    - Steroid
    - Appropriate home medications
- Call House officer on arrival to floor
- Call House officer for (examples): HR < 50 or > 120, SBP < 90 or > 160, T ≥ 38.5, RR > 30, SaO_2 < 90%, UOP < 30 cc/hr, change in exam
- Labs/Studies/Films on arrival, q (frequency), in am

Preop Orders

Diet (e.g., clear liquids until MN)
Bowel prep (if relevant)
Hibiclens shower tonight (or other time)
NPO after MN (or other time)
Void on call to OR (if relevant)
Prep and clip operative site in preop holding (or in am, etc.)
Antibiotic in preop holding
T/S, Crossmatch n units (if indicated)

Bowel Prep (complete) for Colon Surgery

Clear liquid diet for 2 days prior to surgery
Cathartic (one)
- Polyethylene glycol solution (4 L)
- Mag. citrate (240 ml)
- Fleets Phospho-soda
- Mag. sulfate (30 ml) x 3

Topical antibiotic (both)
- Neomycin, 1 g po at 1 pm, 2 pm, and 11 pm
- Erythromycin base, 1 g po (or Metronidazole) at 1 pm, 2 pm, and 11 pm

NPO after MN
Enema (with or without neomycin) – optional

Notes

Preop Note — To be completed before *every* operative case

MR/MRS X is a N-yo M/F with DIAGNOSIS who will undergo PROCEDURE. The diagnosis and treatment options have been discussed with MR/MRS X (or FAMILY OF). HE/SHE understands the benefits and risks, including A, B, and C and wishes to proceed with surgery.

Checklist:

- ☐ Consent
- ☐ Orders
- ☐ Preop antibiotics
- ☐ Lab data
  - Chemistries
  - Hematologic data
  - Coagulation parameters
  - T/S or Type and cross (and units)
  - UA
- ☐ EKG
- ☐ CXR
- ☐ Other studies

Op Note — To be completed after *every* procedure/operative case

Preop Dx:
Postop Dx:
Procedure:
Surgeons:
Assistants:
Anesthesia:
Op findings:
Cross-clamp/Ischemia/Shunt times:
Fluids/Blood Products:
Estimated blood loss (EBL):
UOP:
Drains/Chest tubes:
Specimens:
Cultures:
Complications
Condition:
Disposition/Destination:

Postop Note — To be completed after *every* procedure/operative case

Status post (procedure)
VS: HR BP RR T
Oxygenation: SaO_2 on (form/level of oxygen)
I/O including drain/tube outputs
Physical Exam
- General
- Mental status
- Lungs
- Heart
- Operative site
- Relevant findings (e.g., skin perfusion, pulse, doppler findings, and sensorimotor exam of revascularized limb)

Available lab data
Assessment
Plan

Dictations

Operative Dictation

This is [YOUR NAME] dictating an operative note for Dr. [ATTENDING] on the patient [Patient's NAME and MEDICAL RECORD NUMBER] on [DATE].

Preoperative diagnosis: [PREOP DX],
Postoperative diagnosis: [POSTOP DX],
Procedure(s): [PROCEDURE(S)],

Surgeon(s): [PRIMARY SURGEON(S)],
Assistant(s): [ASSISTANT(S)],
Anesthesia: [TYPE OF ANESTHESIA],
Estimated blood loss (optional): [EBL in cc]
Complications: [NONE, or COMPLICATIONS]
Condition following procedure: [STABLE, or OTHER CONDITION]

Brief clinical note: Mr./Mrs. [PATIENT NAME] is a X-year old male/female with [CONDITION(S), if any], who was evaluated by [DOCTOR] in [CLINIC, or OTHER LOCATION] for [REASON]. [STUDIES] showed [FINDINGS], and [PATIENT] was felt to require [PLAN]. [PATIENT] presents now for [PROCEDURE].

Description of procedure: After informed consent [by POWER OF ATTORNEY OR OTHER LEGAL CONSENTEE, if not patient] and appropriate preoperative evaluation, the patient was taken to the operating room. He/she was placed in [POSITION] and was prepped and draped in the routine fashion for [PROCEDURE]. A [TYPE OF INCISION] was made with [KNIFE/OTHER INSTRUMENT], and.... [FINDINGS]. [PROCEDURE]. All needle, sponge and instrument counts were/were not correct.

The patient was taken to the [POSTOP DESTINATION] [EXTUBATED/INTUBATED] and in [CONDITION]. There were no complications [or list COMPLICATIONS]. Dr. [ATTENDING] was [PRESENT and SCRUBBED, or other participation] for [THE ENTIRE, THE IMPORTANT PORTIONS, or other parts] of the case.

End of dictation

Chapter V

RADIOLOGIC STUDIES

Conventional Radiographs

CXR

Indications: trauma, dyspnea/hypoxia, post-op fever (when feasible, obtain a PA/LAT CXR instead of a portable due to lower cost and better diagnostic info)

Findings:

1. Check tubes and lines (ETT should be 2-5 cm above the carina, CVP line at the cavo-atrial junction)
2. **Edema** — fluffy increased opacity, often associated with hilar fullness
3. **Pulmonary embolus** — findings insensitive and nonspecific. **But always start with CXR!** It may show other cause (edema, pneumonia, PTX), and is required for V/Q scan interpretation. Next step can be V/Q scan or CT, depending upon institution.
4. **Aspiration pneumonitis/pneumonia** — Heterogeneous opacities in posterior lower lobes (a good reason to obtain PA/LAT CXR, not portable!), superior segments of lower lobes in supine pts. Can mimic pulmonary edema
5. **Atelectasis** — increased density, espcially at the lung bases; left lower lobe collapse is common in ICU, especially post-CABG
6. **PTX** — air in the pleura, sourrounding the lung; remember the deep sulcus sign on films obtained with the patient positioned supine (increased lucency at the lung base/in the costophrenic sulcus)
7. **Pneumomediastinum** — air surrounding the bronchus and/or heart can indicate injury to proximal airway (trachea or mainstem bronchi), or esophagus in penetrating trauma (very rare)
8. **Aortic injury** — no finding is sensitive or specific enough to confirm or exclude aortic injury, but radiographic signs suggestive of mediastinal hematoma are listed in Table V.1. Protocols differ by institution, but if one or more of the findings below are present and there is a mechanism for aortic injury, a mediastinal CT scan to evaluate for mediastinal hematoma, or either helical CT or aortography to R/O aortic injury, may be indicated. In trauma pts with a low likelihood of aortic rupture who can tolerate it, upright CXR is safe, cost-effective, and may resolve the question about a mediastinal hematoma suggested by a portable/supine film.

Table V.1. Radiographic Signs of Mediastinal Hematoma
Superior mediastinum > 8 cm wide
Prominence or indistinctness of proximal descending aorta (aortic knob)
Deviation of NGT or ETT/trachea to right (mimicked by pt rotation)
1st–2nd rib, sternal or scapular fx
Left apical cap or left hemothorax
Depression of left main bronchus >140 degrees
Lateral displacement of left paraspinal stripe

KUB/Upright Abd film — Indications: nausea/vomiting, abdominal pain, distension

Findings:

1. **Free air** — Peritoneal air outside the bowel lumen, best seen on upright CXR or KUB but can also be seen on a lateral film (look for air over the lateral margin of the liver). Free retroperitoneal air (e.g., from duodenal perforation) can be loculated. Look for air that does not move; may outline psoas or kidney, thus making those structures more visible.
2. **SBO vs. ileus** — look for air in the colon/rectum, although can still be present with early or partial SBO. Paucity of bowel gas in pt with convincing signs of obstruction may be due to fluid-filled loops. Differentiate a dilated loop as small bowel or colon by location and appearance of folds — thin and circumferential = small bowel (plicae circulares); thick, noncircumferential = colon (haustra). Presence or degree of obstruction can be difficult to predict on KUB alone. Serial KUBs are useful. Findings that favor a high-grade SBO are:
    a. Size of dilated loops (Table V.2), although ileus can yield impressive dilation
    b. Number of dilated loops. Ileus can be focal but is more often diffuse; however a proximal SBO is less confused with ileus than a distal SBO is because only a few jejunal loops may be dilated
    c. Progressively greater bowel dilatation on serial films
    d. Persistent (or progressive) paucity of colonic gas
3. **Pneumatosis intestinalis** — air bubbles within the bowel wall, concern for ischemia
4. **Assorted calcifications**
    a. RUQ — Gallstones, plain film has very poor sensitivity since most are not radiopaque
    b. Pancreas — Chronic pancreatitis
    c. Kidney stones — Spiral CT has replaced KUB/IVP due to superior sensitivity and specificity and decreased need for IV contrast
    d. Appendicolith — Insensitive but specific for appendicitis when present

e. Splenic — Common and incidental, usually from prior infection or trauma
f. Vascular — Tubular, most dramatic in renal and diabetic pts

Table V.2. Maximum Normal Caliber of Bowel Loops In Adults	
Small bowel	3 cm
Cecum	9 cm
Transverse colon	6 cm

Ultrasound

Note: There are generally no contraindications to US, but morbidly obese pts can render interpretation more difficult.

FAST [43]

(Focused Assessment with Sonography for the evaluation of Trauma):

Indications: evaluation of intraperitoneal fluid/blood in unstable or pregnant trauma pts

Prep: None.

Description: Search for free fluid/hemoperitoneum (fluid appears black on US) in the following locations: **Pericardial, Perihepatic, Perisplenic, Pelvic** (four Ps). This is **not** a good modality to look for organ-specific injuries or retroperitoneal hemorrhage.

Pitfalls:
1. Pre-existing liver failure/ascites
2. Peritoneal dialysis
3. DPL at previous hospital (if you are working at a referral trauma center)
4. Fluid in bowel loops
5. Small amount of fluid in cul-de-sac can be normal in menstruation or pregnancy
6. Technique — factors such as gain settings and room lighting can dramatically alter the sensitivity of US

Gallbladder/Biliary US

Prep: Avoid narcotics until after study. Should be NPO for 4-6 hrs to distend GB

Indications: RUQ or epigastric pain/tenderness, fever, laboratory evidence of cholestasis, suspected complication of cholecystectomy or biliary tract procedure

Findings:

1. **Gallstones** — US is more sensitive than CT
2. **Sonographic Murphy's sign** — Pain/inspiratory cessation upon US guided compression of the gallbladder. This is regarded as more specific than Murphy's sign on physical exam, since GB is directly visualized. US has high positive predictive value if both gallstones and this sign are observed, and even better negative predictive value if both are absent (sensitivity and specificity >95%)
3. Other findings (**GB wall thickening, pericholecystic fluid, enlarged GB** [Table V.3]) are suggestive but not as sensitive or specific

Table V.3. Normal Biliary Tract Measurements

GB wall thickness	GB max size	CBD size
Up to 3 mm	5 x 10 cm	6 mm, can be larger over age 60 or after cholecystectomy

Carotid US

Indications: Screening of pts at high risk, stroke, bruit (controversial)

Prep: None

What to look for:
Degree of stenosis is estimated based on Doppler velocity measurements (Table V.4). When measurements do not yield a consistent degree of stenosis, correlation is made with the appearance on color Doppler imaging to give an estimated degree of stenosis.

Table V.4. Carotid Doppler Velocity Measurements

% stenosis	Peak systolic velocity	Peak diastolic velocity	Systolic velocity ICA/CCA ratio	Diastolic velocity ICA/CCA ratio
0–39	< 110	< 40	< 1.8	< 2.4
40–59	110–130	40	< 1.8	< 2.4
60–79	130–250	41–100	1.8–3.7	2.4–5.5
80–99	> 250	> 100	> 3.7	> 5.5

Pitfall:
A very high-grade stenosis may appear occluded on US. In any pt with carotid occlusion by US, one should consider a carotid angiogram to exclude a very high-grade stenosis (often requiring surgery in the latter case). MRA often cannot make this distinction.

RLQ US

Ultrasound is reported as 85–95% accurate in diagnosing appendicitis, is most often used in children (smaller body habitus conducive to US) and menstrual-age females (US can evaluate right ovary/adnexa better than CT scan)

Computed Tomography

The Use of Contrast Agents
The need for oral or IV contrast depends on the indication:
1. IV contrast actually lowers the sensitivity for detecting **renal or ureteral stones**.
2. IV and oral contrast are not needed for **retroperitoneal bleeding** (e.g., leaking AAA), and will only delay the time to diagnosis (note: *rupture* mandates emergent surgery, rather than CT scan); but IV contrast is crucial in the evaluation of aortic dissection.
3. **Most centers** administer enteral contrast for trauma CT or evaluating intestinal obstruction.
4. Protocols to **R/O appendicitis** vary, from oral, rectal and IV to rectal only or no contrast at all.

Consult radiologist regarding the need for IV, oral or rectal/stomal contrast when requesting a study, especially if you are unsure. This may change how you prepare the pt:
1. Will pt require an **NGT** for enteral contrast (if unable to take p.o.)?
2. Does pt have a **contrast/iodine/shellfish allergy**? If so, can the study wait for a **steroid prep** (4–24 hrs)? If not, is there an alternative (noncontrast CT, MRI, US, nuclear medicine studies)?
3. Does the pt need **rectal contrast**? If needed, this will usually be administered by the radiologist. But if pt has a recent rectal or anal anastomosis, your assistance/approval is necessary.
4. Does pt have **adequate IV access** for contrast? **Central lines,** especially **PICC lines,** generally will not be used for this, particularly certain studies that require boluses injected as a rapid bolus (CT angiogram, pulmonary embolism).
5. Check patient's **creatinine** — cutoff may vary, generally must be ≤ 2.0 (unless on dialysis). Depending on indication, MRI may be an alternative since gadolinium (MR contrast) is not nephrotoxic. If IV contrast is given to a marginal patient, be certain pt is well hydrated.

Head CT

Indications: Head trauma, altered mental status or neurological exam

Prep: None. Contrast not needed for most acute indications. Exceptions include r/o mets or brain abscess, HIV pts, CT angiogram to r/o dissection or aneurysm.

Trauma
Findings:

1. Blood — Acute blood appears more dense (brighter) than brain parenchyma on CT. The density decreases with age of blood and lower pt hematocrit.
   a. **Epidural hematoma** classically has a lentiform (lens-shaped) appearance, and is limited in its spread by the skull sutures but not dural reflections (tentorium, falx). Traumatic epidural hematomas usually result from injury to the middle meningeal artery, although temporal bone fracture may not be present. Due to the (usually) arterial source and potential for rapid herniation, this is a true emergency, neurosurgery should be consulted immediately.
   b. **Subdural hematoma** is usually crescentic in shape, limited by dural reflections but not sutures. Source is usually venous (cortical veins). More often bilateral than epidural hematoma. Less frequently requires surgery, depends on degree of mass effect.
   c. **Subarachnoid** — blood in CSF cisterns, fissures, ventricles.
   d. **Parenchymal** — contusion (frontal, anterior temporal), shear injury (gray-white junction, basal ganglia, corpus callosum). Shear injury may not manifest immediately on CT scan since it results in petechial bleeds, may account for low GCS that is not explained by CT findings. Some MRI sequences are more sensitive for this, may be needed for prognostic or legal purposes.
2. **Cerebral edema** — loss of the normal distinction between gray and white matter, effacement of normal CSF spaces (cisterns, sulci, ventricles). Can be difficult to identify in young children, since brain appears tightly packed in normal infants.
3. **Fracture** — CT excels at detecting fx. Types of fractures:
   a. Orbital floor/maxillary sinus roof — can be easily missed on axial images. Look for blood in maxillary sinus, entrapment of inferior rectus muscle (clinical), obtain direct or reconstructed coronal imaging as fx is much easier to visualize.
   b. Medial orbital wall — thin rim of bone separating orbit from ethmoid sinus is the lamina papyracea, and as name implies is easily fractured. Look for intraorbital air, blood in ethmoids.
   c. Lower temporal bone — may have concomitant facial nerve injury.
   d. Skull base — increased risk of carotid dissection or carotid-cavernous sinus fistula.

Stroke

Findings of acute stroke can be subtle or absent. With continued evolution of the role of thrombolytic therapy, it is imperative to obtain a head CT to R/O ICH. Even in absence of CT findings, acute stroke remains a clinical diagnosis and pt may be a candidate for thrombolysis if no bleed is present. Always call for an emergent head CT as soon as stroke is suspected.

Body CT

Indications: Myriad — trauma, abscess, malignancy, AAA, bowel obstruction, PE, others.

Prep: See above re: **Contrast**.

Findings:

1. **Trauma** — not all centers give oral contrast (see above).
   a. Major visceral injuries — spleen, liver, kidney are common. Pancreatic injury can be subtle — look for linear hypodensity through neck or proximal body (overlying the spine). Right adrenal hemorrhage is much more common than left.
   b. Unexplained mesenteric fluid/blood may be the only finding in traumatic bowel injury; extraluminal oral contrast or air is uncommon even with transected bowel.
   c. Chest — Many surgeons recommend aortography in the evaluation of all mediastinal hematomas. Some recent studies suggest that helical CT findings of aortic injury (flap, extraluminal contrast, irregular wall) may have adequate sensitivity and specificity (both > 99%) for use as the definitive diagnostic modality in this setting.[40,41]
2. **Abscess** — oral and IV contrast preferred, rectal may be needed in cases of diverticulitis or appendicitis.
   a. Oral contrast helps distinguish bowel from abscess.
   b. IV contrast shows rim-enhancement, distinguishing abscess from free fluid. Also highlights mesenteric vessels and hence may alter approach to percutaneous drainage.
3. **Pulmonary embolus** — CT has rapidly gained favor as the diagnostic study of choice at many centers. Although no truly randomized studies have compared CT to the conventional algorithm (V/Q, then angio if needed), some studies suggest that a negative CT for PE is highly specific for no adverse outcome from PE. Also, CT can more sensitively evaluate the parenchyma than CXR (e.g., edema, aspiration, early infection). But if your pt has non-dialysis–dependent renal insufficiency, contrast allergy or no usable IV for injection, you may need to obtain V/Q. Criteria, availability and preference for CT vs V/Q may vary by institution and physician; always check with your radiologist and senior resident/staff.
4. **CT angiography** — has replaced angiography at some centers. Common uses include evaluation of AAA, aortic dissection, mesenteric/splenic pseudoaneurysm, preoperative evaluation of renal arteries in living-related kidney donor.

GI (Luminal) Radiology

Types of Contrast Agents:

Swallow

1. Barium (or other contrast) swallow is designed to examine the esophagus from pharynx to GE junction, usually for tumor, stricture, dysmotility/reflux, anastomotic leak or rupture. (Alternatively, a speech swallow assesses the swallowing mechanism from mouth to proximal esophagus to determine aspiration risk. This is usually performed in conjunction with a speech pathologist, and may require a consult to speech path prior to obtaining it.)
2. Let radiologist know the indication. Most inpatients or ER pts will be to r/o obstruction, rupture or anastomotic leak, and will be performed with single water-soluble contrast technique.
3. Sensitivity for esophageal perforation/leak is improved by performing gastrograffin *followed* by barium study if the former study is negative. The reason for performing the gastrograffin study first is to avoid leakage of a significant amount of barium into the mediastium in the event of a large leak, as barium may cause severe inflammation. Gastrograffin, however, is poorly tolerated by the lungs, and therefore barium should be used if there is a significant risk of aspiration in a particular patient. Similar concerns apply to the use of contrast in any part of the GI tract (UGI/SBFT/BE), as barium can cause severe inflammation in the peritoneal cavity, as well.
4. **Prep:** Emergent study requires no prep. Keep NPO after midnight for elective study (usually not a problem since the purpose for most will be to check a fresh anastomosis, and pts may be on TPN or j-tube feeds).

Upper GI — Studies the GI track from proximal esophagus to duodenum. **Prep** is usually NPO after midnight.

Small bowel follow-through/enteroclysis

1. Make sure you know which one you need, as these are distinctly different exams. SBFT involves ingestion of PO contrast, with serial radiographs until contrast reaches colon. Directed fluoroscopy is performed as needed, such as at possible transition points in obstruction or the terminal ileum in Crohn's disease. Enteroclysis, or small bowel enema, involves advancing a tube into the distal duodenum/proximal jejunum, and administering contrast and a distending agent (methylcellulose). This provides more mucosal detail, but is more uncomfortable and associated with added risk. Consult your attending and radiologist to clarify which one is needed and safe.
2. **Prep:** Varies depending on indication and which study is ordered. Check with radiology department as soon as you order the study.
3. Normal transit time to cecum is 2 hours.

Barium/Gastrograffin enema

1. This ranges from a limited single contrast study to r/o sigmoid volvulus, to complete air-contrast barium enema exam of the entire colon to look for polyp/tumor.
2. **Prep** ranges from none (volvulus, obstruction, leak), to extensive colonic cleansing beginning the morning prior to day of exam (polyp search). Consult radiology as soon as you order an enema, especially if double-contrast exam is requested.

Nuclear Medicine

V/Q Scan — Despite the emergence of CT for detecting PE, this remains a well-established tool. There are generally no contraindications for V/Q, all the pt needs is some kind of IV access. Even if your center prefers CT, V/Q will be your study of choice if pt is not a CT candidate (see #3 above under **Body CT** and **Contrast**, both under **Computed Tomography**).

HIDA Scan — Used to diagnose acute cholecystitis by demonstrating cystic duct obstruction. Intravenous radiotracer is taken up by the liver and excreted into bile. A positive HIDA is defined as tracer clearly present in small bowel via the common bile duct, with no GB visualization 1 hr after SB seen. GB visualization at any time constitutes a negative HIDA.

1. ICU and TPN pts can have biliary stasis, requiring delayed imaging (up to 24 hrs).
2. **Prep: Do not give narcotics or food** to any pt who may need a HIDA scan. Narcotics may result in delayed or absent appearance of tracer in CBD/GB from increased sphincter of Oddi tone. Recent meal causes GB contraction, which can result in a false positive HIDA.
3. Hepatocyte dysfunction (e.g. hepatitis), cholestasis and acute CBD obstruction can result in decreased or absent tracer excretion, limiting the specificity of a nonvisualized GB in these settings.

Tagged RBC Scan — For localization of GI bleeding; requires active bleeding at 0.05-0.4 ml/min to yield positive study.

1. Usually required prior to angiography, since this test is more sensitive (angio shows active bleeding at 1 ml/min, and must be ongoing when contrast is injected), and clinical evidence of bleeding (melena/hematochezia, hemodynamic changes) can manifest after bleeding has stopped.
2. Tagged RBC scan is not as reliable for upper GI bleeding, since free pertechnetate (tracer unincorporated by RBC) is excreted by gastric mucosa.
3. Generally **no prep needed**, although upper GI source should be excluded by gastric lavage prior to ordering scan.

PET Scan — Rapidly evolving modality used primarily in diagnosing and staging malignancy. It exploits the hypermetabolic state of tumor cells. A radiolabeled glucose analog is given intravenously, pt rests quietly for 30–45 minutes and is then imaged, with "hot" areas indicating elevated cellular metabolism and possible malignancy.

1. **Prep:** Pt must be NPO for 4 hrs (to keep insulin level low, otherwise too much tracer goes to skeletal muscle).
2. Diabetics should have glucose control optimized before injection. Generally, a blood sugar of 200 or less is desired to achieve reasonable distribution of tracer.

Magnetic Resonance Imaging

General information:
MRI has many uses, most often, but not limited to, neurologic, musculoskeletal and vascular imaging. Advantages of MRI over CT include non-nephrotoxic contrast, flow-sensitive imaging and increased tissue characterization. Disadvantages include a variety of artifacts, cost, availability, and lengthy study times.

Patients are carefully screened by radiology personnel prior to entering the magnet area. Common exclusion criteria:

1. A **pacemaker** is an **absolute contraindication** to MRI.
2. Patients with a history of orbital **metallic foreign body** need radiographs or CT to determine if residual metal is present.
3. Many surgical prosthetics and hardware do not prohibit MRI, but may degrade image quality. Ask your radiologist; know what pt has, how long it has been there, and what you want imaged.
4. **Claustrophobic** pts and children may need sedation.
5. MRI contrast (gadolinium) is not nephrotoxic, although your center may have a maximum creatinine cutoff for its use.

Vascular/Interventional Radiology

General information:
When requesting an intervention from radiology, there are basic principles common to most procedures.

1. **Consent** — This should generally be performed by the radiologist, who knows the technique and risks better than you. In some cases, he/she may ask for your help (emergency consent, family contact if pt unconsentable).
2. **Bleeding diathesis —** Acceptable values for platelets, PT, and PTT vary by type of procedure (e.g., fistulogram vs. TIPS), clinical urgency, and consulting radiologist.

3. **Allergies**
   a. Iodine/contrast/shellfish? If so, what was the reaction? Steroid prep may be required, especially if study can wait 12–24 hrs. Some studies do not require iodinated contrast (such as most biopsies), others can be performed with alternative agents (CO_2, gadolinium). If allergy is life-threatening, consider other options (MRA instead of angio, ERCP or MRCP instead of PTC).
   b. Sedatives or local anesthetics — commonly used in radiology.
4. **Renal function** — Serum creatinine only important for intravascular contrast (GU and biliary procedures generally do not require this, except for TIPS). Consider alternative studies if serum creat > 2.0; if unavailable and situation is urgent, risk of possible renal damage (temporary or permanent) may need to be accepted, or alternative contrast agents (gadolinium or CO_2) are used at some centers. This should be mentioned during consent.
5. **NPO** — in general, required if sedation to be used. When in doubt, keep NPO. Even simple procedures are poorly tolerated by some pts with low pain threshold.

Angiography

General Information

1. **Sedation** generally used, keep pt NPO.
2. **Know** and **explain** what information you are looking for and what your plan is before the procedure begins. Examples —
   a. Do you want both lower extremities or just one?
   b. If obtaining a trauma arch aortogram, is there a diminished extremity pulse, thus requiring directed injection(s)?
   c. Do you want angioplasty/stent if pt is a candidate?
   d. For GI bleeding, do you want the GDA coiled even if diagnostic study is negative in pt with upper GI bleed? Do you want a heparin challenge?
3. Pulses — for extremities, absent femoral pulses may necessitate a brachial artery approach. This is especially important to know if intervention is planned, since larger access is needed for stent/angioplasty and vascular surgery assistance may be required for doing this via the upper extremity.
4. **Pulmonary angiography** — May only be performed selectively at your center if CT is used to diagnose PE. Obtain EKG to look for left bundle branch block. Transient right bundle block can occur during this procedure, resulting in complete block if LBBB exists. Radiologist may want external pacer placed prior to procedure in this case.

Angioplasty/Stent Placement

Patients may ask you questions about angioplasty/stenting. While you should defer most of these to the interventionist, a basic knowledge of success and patency rates may be handy. With continued evolution of stent materials, antiplatelet agent use, and possibly even intravascular pharmacological or gene therapy, patency rates are likely to improve.

1. **Iliac angioplasty** is technically successful in about 90% of pts, > 95% with stenting.
   a. 4- to 5-year patency ~ 95% with stent, 70% with angioplasty alone.
   b. Major complication (arterial rupture, dissection that compromises flow, distal embolization) occurs in <3%. About 1% require surgery.
   c. Acute restenosis may occur in 1–2% without stenting, less often with stenting. Causes are thrombosis, spasm, elastic recoil.
2. **Femoral/popliteal angioplasty** has technical success rate of ~ 95%. Stents are generally not deployed below the inguinal ligament at this time, except if needed to manage complications (such as major dissection).
   a. One-year patency is 60–80%.
   b. Reported five-year patency rates range widely from ~ 15–60%, but rates for pts with short-segment stenosis and good runoff (50–60%) compare favorably to 5-yr patency of surgical fem-pop bypass (50–75%).
3. **Renal angioplasty and stenting**
   a. Indications include renovascular hypertension that is refractory to medical management, and/or deteriorating renal function.
   b. Clinical results are better for fibromuscular dysplasia than atherosclerosis.
   c. MRA is a good screening study for pts with suspected renal artery stenosis, especially due to non-nephrotoxic contrast.
4. **Percutaneously deployed aortic stent grafts** have shown great promise in select pts. Stent graft design, criteria for their use, and clinical experience are rapidly evolving.

IVC filter Placement — Filters are placed for those who are at high risk for or have known DVT's and for whom anticoagulation is contraindicated (e.g., head injured patients). Know the site of documented DVT. Preferred access sites are right common femoral vein and right internal jugular vein. See general information above, since contrast is generally used to assure infrarenal deployment of filter and document size of IVC.

Percutaneous Drains

1. Most drains, including PCNs and PBDs, should be regularly flushed with 5–10 cc of sterile saline 2-3 times a day to prevent clogging. The radiologist will generally write orders for this; if you are not certain, call the radiologist.

2. If drain output slows or stops, think of the possibilities:
   a. Drain is clogged — flush it and see.
   b. Abscess has resolved — pull drain or obtain CT to confirm.
   c. Drain has migrated or been inadvertently pulled back — note how much tubing is outside body. If this is suspected, imaging may be required (fluoroscopy or CT).
3. Transient bacteremia and fever are common after PBD placement.
4. Abdominal abscesses, postoperative or not, are now commonly drained percutaneously by radiologists under US or CT guidance. Even if CT is used, contrast typically is unnecessary for the actual drainage.
5. Pleural drainage — radiologist may require evidence that pleural fluid is infected or malignant prior to drain placement.

Biopsy

1. See general information above. While contrast may have been used for the diagnostic CT, contrast is generally not required for CT-guided biopsy. No ultrasound contrast agent is currently in widespread clinical use.
2. Do not specifically request CT or US guidance; the radiologist will decide which is appropriate.
3. Have pt's films reviewed and procedure approved by radiologist prior to day of biopsy.
4. If infection is a diagnostic consideration, specifically request that material for culture be obtained.

Hemodialysis Access

1. When requesting dialysis catheter placement, know pt's hemodialysis access/central venous catheter hx: location of prior catheters and fistulas/grafts, time most recent one was removed or malfunctioned and why (infected, occluded, fistula matured, renal function returned, transplant), the plan regarding future permanent hemodialysis access (indwelling catheter predisposes to venous stenosis, new catheter should be placed to avoid extremity where fistula is planned if feasible).
2. **Fistulogram/plasty/lysis** — This is an alternative to surgical revision of a dialysis graft, with variable results. Know age and history of prior interventions on current fistula. Know if you would like a hemodialysis catheter placed if plasty/lysis depending on technical success. If so, above info applies.

APPENDICES

Appendix A: Abbreviations

aa	Arteries
AAA	Abdominal aortic aneurysm
Abd	Abdominal/abdomen
ABG	Arterial blood gas
ADAT	Advance diet as tolerated
A-gram	Arteriogram
AIDS	Acquired immunodeficiency syndrome
AK	Above-knee
AKA	Above-knee amputation
A-line	Arterial line
alt	Alternatively
amp	Ampule
Appy	Appendectomy
ARF	Acute renal failure
AS	Aortic stenosis
ASIS	Anterior superior iliac spine
AV	Arteriovenous
AVF	Arteriovenous fistula
BI	Billroth I gastric reconstruction
BII	Billroth II gastric reconstruction
BCx	Blood cultures
bid	Twice a day
BKA	Below-knee amputation
BP	Blood pressure
C	Camera (laparoscope)
C&S	Culture & Sensitivities (bacterial)
CA	Cancer
CABG	Coronary artery bypass grafting
CAD	Coronary artery disease
CAPD	Chronic ambulatory peritoneal dialysis
CBC	Complete blood count
CBD	Common bile duct
CEA	Carotid endarterectomy
CFA	Common femoral artery
CHF	Congestive heart failure
CI	Common iliac
CIA	Common iliac artery
CIV	Common iliac vein
CO	Cardiac output
Complics	Complications

Contralat.	Contralateral
Controv.	Controversial
COPD	Chronic obstructive pulmonary disease
CPB	Cardiopulmonary bypass
CRF	Chronic renal failure
CXR	Chest X-ray
D_{50}	Glucose, 50% solution in water (50 g/100 ml)
D1, D2, etc.	First portion of the duodenum, second portion, etc.
D/C	Discharge, or Discontinue
DBP	Diastolic blood pressure
DHT	Dobhoff tube
Diam.	Diameter
DIC	Disseminated intravascular coagulation
DM	Diabetes mellitus
d/o	Disorder
Drsg	Dressing
Dx	Diagnosis
Dz	Disease
ECA	External carotid artery
EEA	End-to-end anastomosis (stapler)
esp	Especially
fr	French (circumference in millimeters)
F/U	Follow-up
GB	Gallbladder
G-tube	Gastrostomy tube
G-E	Gastroesophageal
GYN	Gynecologic
Hct	Hematocrit
HR	Heart rate
Hx	History
IAPT	Ileoanal pull-through
ICA	Internal carotid artery
ICH	Intracranial hemorrhage
IJ	Internal jugular vein
IM	Intramuscularly
IMA	Inferior mesenteric artery
IMV	Inferior mesenteric vein
Indic	Indication
Ipsilat.	Ipsilateral
IS	Incentive spirometry
IV	Intravenous
IVA	IV analgesia
IVC	Inferior vena cava
JP	Jackson-Pratt (closed suction) drain
J-tube	Jejunostomy tube
LOT	Ligament of Treitz
LWS	Low wall suction
MAC	Monitored anesthesia care (local anesthesia with sedation

	per anesthesia)
MAP	Mean arterial pressure
MN	Midnight
MODS	Multi-organ dysfunction syndrome (a.k.a., multi-organ failure)
MR	Mitral regurgitation
MRA	Magnetic resonance angiography
MRM	Modified radical mastectomy
NGT	Nasogastric tube
NJT	Nasojejunal tube
NTG	Nitroglycerin
NPO	Nothing per os
N/V	Nausea and vomiting
OGT	Orogastric tube
P.	Pectoralis (major or minor)
PBD	Percutaneous biliary drain
PCA	Patient-controlled anesthesia
PCN	Percutaneous nephrostomy tube
PCP	*Pneumocystis carinii* pneumonia
PE	Pulmonary embolus
PEG	Percutaneous endoscopic gastrostomy
PET	Positron emission tomography
PEx	Physical exam
PFA	Profunda femoris artery
PFT	Pulmonary function testing
Pheo	Pheochromocytoma
PLT	Platelet count
PO	Per os (by mouth)
Popliteal	Popliteal artery
Posn	Position
Postop	Postoperative management
PPW	Pylorus-preserving Whipple
Preop	Preoperative assessment
Proc	Procedure
Prox	Proximal
Pulm	Pulmonary
Pt	Patient
PT	Prothrombin time
PTFE	Polytetrafluoroethylene
PTT	Partial thromboplastin time
PVD	Peripheral vascular disease
Qac	Before meals
Qhs	At bedtime (hour of sleep)
RA	Right atrium
RAS	Renal artery stenosis
Relat	Relationship
RLN	Recurrent laryngeal nerve
R/O	Rule out
RR	Respiratory rate

RSVG	Reversed saphenous vein graft
Rx	Treatment
SaO_2	Arterial oxygen saturation
SB	Small bowel
SBO	Small bowel obstruction
SBP	Systolic blood pressure
SC	Subclavian vein
SCDs	Sequential compression devices
SCM	Sternocleidomastoid muscle
SFA	Superficial femoral artery
Sgy	Surgery
SMA	Superior mesenteric artery
SNP	Sodium nitroprusside
SubQ	Subcutaneously, or subcutaneous tissue
SV	Saphenous vein
SVC	Superior vena cava
SVG	Saphenous vein graft
T	Temperature
TAPP	Transabdominal preperitoneal
T-burg	Trendelenburg
TIA	Transient ischemic attack
tid	Three times a day
TME	Total mesorectal excision
TOA	Tuboovarian abscess
T/S	Type and screen
Tx	Therapy, Transfer, or Transplant
UA	Urinalysis
UOP	Urine output
UTI	Urinary tract infection
W/U	Work-up
5	5 mm trocar site
10	10 mm trocar site
10C	10 mm trocar site for camera
√	Evaluate
?	Question of

Appendix B: Patient Education Anatomic Drawings

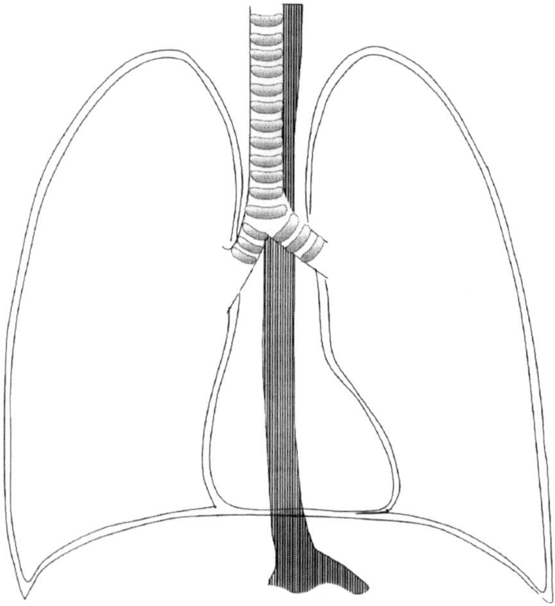

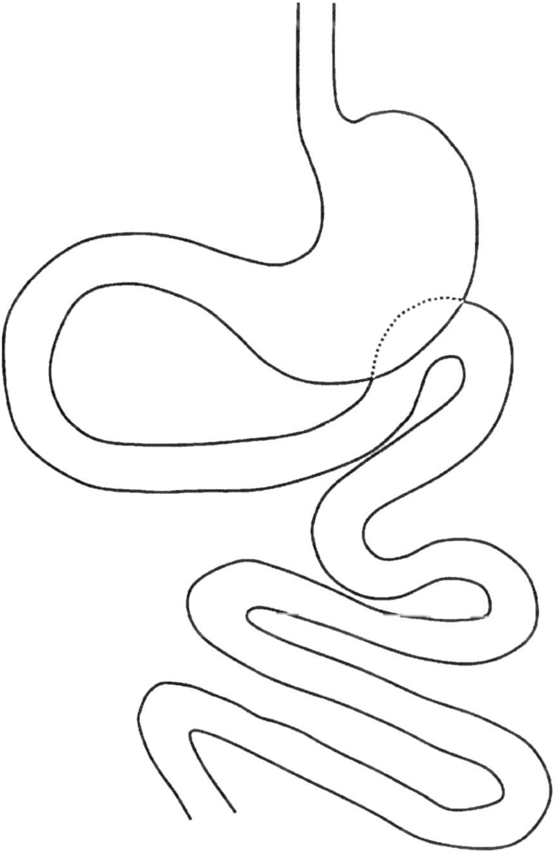

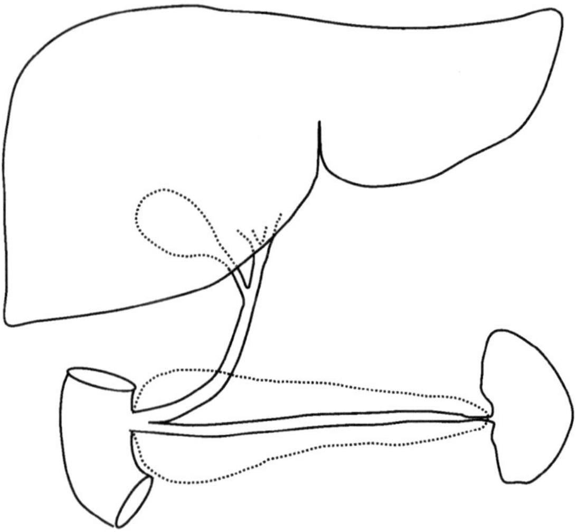

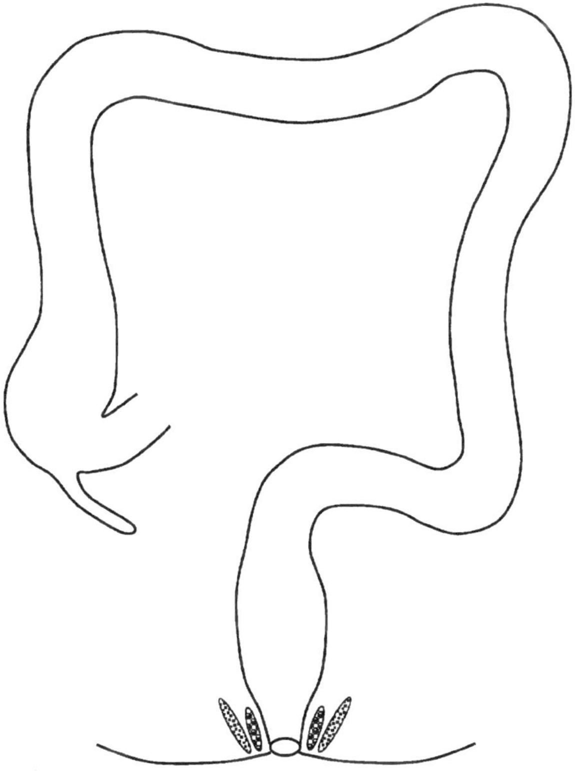

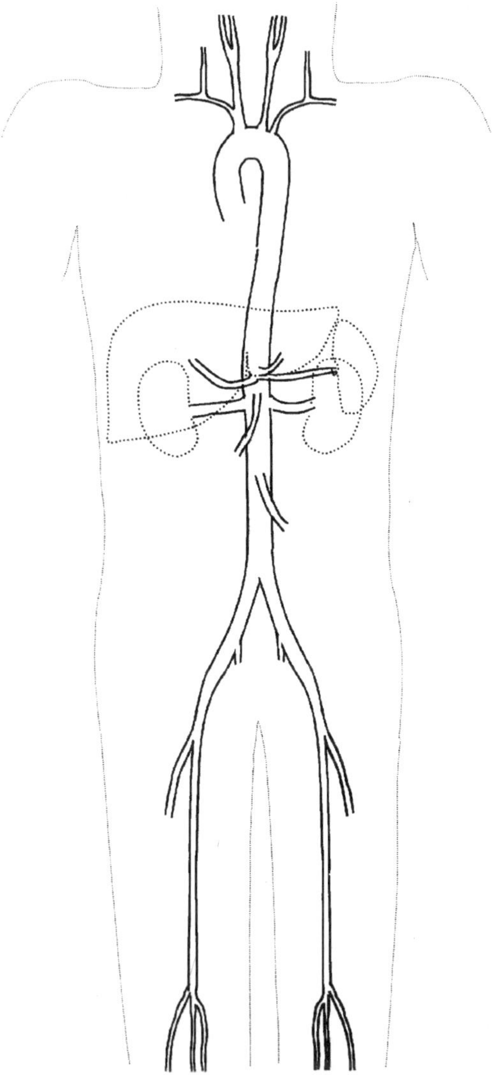

Appendix C: Scales for Measurement

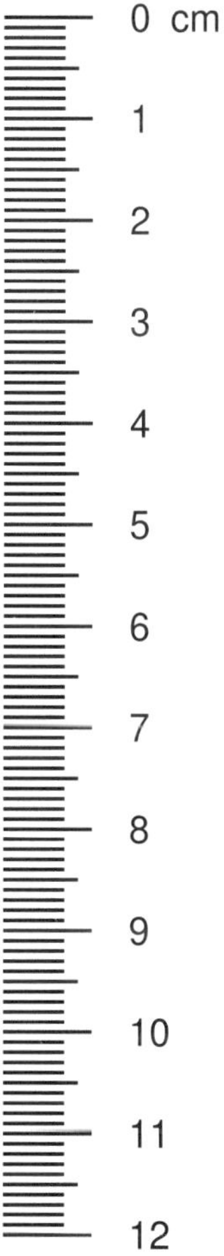

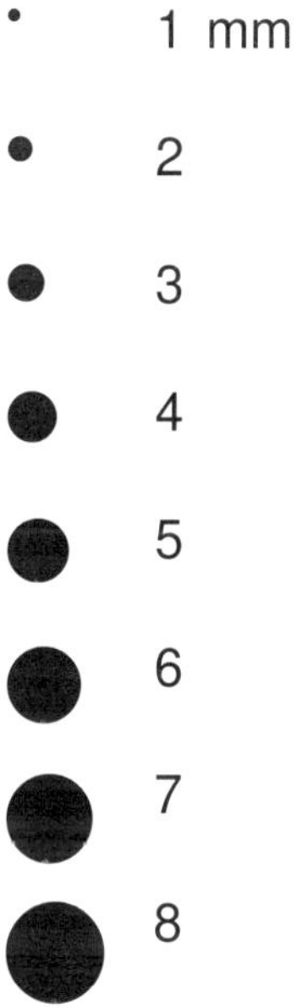

References

1. Janning SW, Rybak MJ. Antimicrobial prophylaxis in surgery. In: DiPiro JT, Talbert RL, Yee GC et al., eds. *Pharmacotherapy*, 4th Edition. Stamford: Appleton and Lange, 1999, pp. 1888–99.
2. Abramowics MA, ed. Antimicrobial prophylaxis in surgery. *The Medical Letter on Drugs and Therapeutics* 41:75-80, 1999.
3. Durack DT. Drug Therapy: Prevention of Infective Endocarditis. *NEJM* 332:38-44, 1995.
4. Skandalakis JE, Skandalakis PN, Skandalakis LJ. *Surgical Anatomy and Technique*, 2nd Edition. New York: Springer, 2000.
5. Lodge AJ, Eubanks S. Laparoscopic adrenalectomy. In: Pappas TN, Chekan EG, Eubanks S, eds. *Atlas of Laparoscopic Surgery*, 2nd Edition. Philadelphia: Current Medicine, 1999, pp. 18.1–9.
6. Smith CD, Weber CJ, Anderson JR. Laparoscopic adrenalectomy: New gold standard. *World Journal of Surgery* 23:389-396, 1999.
7. Tucker JG, Ramshaw BJ. In: Eubanks WS, Swanstrom LL, Soper NJ, eds. *Mastery of Endoscopic and Laparoscopic Surgery*. Philadelphia: Lippincott Williams and Wilkins, 2000, pp. 355–63.
8. Zollinger RMJ, Zollinger RM. *Atlas of Surgical Operations* 7th Edition. New York: McGraw-Hill, 1993.
9. Bergamini T, Taber S, Hoch J. Long-term venous access. In: Rutherford R, ed. *Vascular Surgery*, 5th Edition. Philadelphia: W.B. Saunders, 2000.
10. Daniels LJ, Chekan EG. Laparoscopic cholecystectomy. In: Pappas TN, Chekan EG, Eubanks S, eds. *Atlas of Laparoscopic Surgery*, 2nd Edition. Philadelphia: Current Medicine, 1999, pp. 13.1–13.19.
11. Inculet RI. Transhiatal Esophagectomy. In: Kaiser LR, Kron IL, Spray TL, eds. *Mastery of Cardiothoracic Surgery.* Philadelphia: Lippincott-Raven, 1998, pp. 134–40.
12. Casson AG. Thoracic approaches to esophagectomy. In: Kaiser LR, Kron IL, Spray TL, eds. *Mastery of Cardiothoracic Surgery.* Philadelphia: Lippincott-Raven, 1998, pp. 141–50.
13. Conter R, Kauffman G. Benign Gastric Ulcer and Stress Gastritis. In: Cameron J, ed. *Current Surgical Therapy*, 6th Edition. St. Louis: Mosby, 1995, pp. 75-78.
14. Pappas T. The Stomach and Duodenum: Historical aspects, anatomy, pathology, physiology, and peptic ulcer disease. In: Sabiston DC Jr, Lyerly HK, eds. Textbook of Surgery: *The Biological Basis of Modern Surgical Practice*, 15th Edition. Philidelphia: W.B. Saunders, 1997, pp. 847–868.
15. Watters VA, Grant JP, Fulkerson WJ. *Physician's Guide to Establishing Enteral and Central Venous Access: Unpublished handbook*, 1998.

16. Meyers, WC. Major hepatic resection. In: Sabiston DC Jr, Lyerly HK, eds. *Textbook of Surgery: The Biological Basis of Modern Surgical Practice*, 15th Edition. Philidelphia: W.B. Saunders, 1997, pp. 1082–3.
17. Akhter SA, Eubanks S. Laparoscopic inguinal herniorrhaphy. In: Pappas TN, Chekan EG, Eubanks S, eds. *Atlas of Laparoscopic Surgery*, 2nd Edition. Philadelphia: Current Medicine, 1999, pp. 3.1–3.14.
18. Grant JP. Repair of incisional hernias. In: Sabiston DC Jr, Lyerly HK, eds. *Textbook of Surgery: The Biological Basis of Modern Surgical Practice*, 15th Edition. Philidelphia: W.B. Saunders, 1997, pp. 174–85.
19. Clark LA, Grant JP. Laparoscopic ostomies. In: Pappas TN, Chekan EG, Eubanks S, eds. *Atlas of Laparoscopic Surgery*, 2nd Edition. Philadelphia: Current Medicine, 1999, pp. 9.1–9.8.
20. Weinerth JL. Kidney transplanation. In: Sabiston DC, ed. *Atlas of General Surgery*. Philadelphia: W. B. Saunders, 1994, pp. 683–97.
21. Barker CF, Naji A, Markmann JF, et al. Renal transplanation. In: Sabiston DC, Lyerly HK, eds. *Textbook of Surgery: The Biological Basis of Modern Surgical Practice*, 15th Edition. Philadelphia: W. B. Saunders, 1997, pp. 408–28.
22. Henry ML, Ferguson RM. Renal transplantation. In: Greenfield LJ, Mulholland M, Oldham KT, et al, eds. *Surgery: Scientific Principles and Practice*, 2nd Edition. Philadelphia: Lippincott-Raven, 1997, pp. 571–80.
23. Atkins B, Pappas T. Laparoscopic antireflux procedures. In: Pappas TN, Chekan EG, Eubanks S, eds. *Atlas of Laparoscopic Surgery*, 2nd Edition. Philadelphia: Current Medicine, 1999, pp. 5.1–5.16.
24. Richardson S, Hunter J. Laparoscopic Nissen Fundoplication. In: Cameron J, ed. *Current Surgical Therapy*, 6th Edition. St. Louis: Mosby, 1998.
25. Martin X, Cloix P, Dawahra M, et al. Multiple organ procurement. In: Collins GM, Dubernard JM, Land W, Persijn GG, eds. *Procurement, preservation, and allocation of vascularized organs*. Dordrecht: Kluwer Academic Publishers, 1997.
26. Kaufman DB. Pancreas Transplantation. In: Stuart FP, Abecassis MM, Kaufman DB, eds. *Organ Transplantation*. Georgetown, Tx: Landes Bioscience. 2000, pp. 145–168.
27. Gruessner, A.C., Sutherland, D.E.R. Analyses of Pancreas Transplantation Outcomes for United States Cases Reported to The United Network for Organ Sharing (UNOS) and Non-US Cases Reported to the International Pancreas Transplant Registry (IPTR). In: Cecka JM, Terasaki PI, eds. *Clinical Transplants 1999*, 15th Edition. Los Angeles, CA: UCLA Tissue Typing Laboratory, 2000, pp. 51–69.
28. Stickel DL. Insertion of Tenckhoff catheter. In: Sabiston DCJ, ed. *Atlas of General Surgery*. Philadelphia: W. B. Saunders, 1994, pp. 99–101.
29. Mattei P, Sola JE. Gastrointestinal procedures. In: Chen H, Lillemoe KD, Sola JE, eds. *Manual of Common Bedside Surgical Procedures*. Baltimore: Williams and Wilkins, 1996, pp. 132–63.

30. Farooq M, Freischlag J. Peritoneal Dialysis. In: Rutherford R, ed. *Vascular Surgery*, 5th Edition. Philadelphia: W.B. Saunders, 2000.
31. Grillo HC, Mathisen DJ. Tracheostomy and its complications. In: Sabiston DCJ, Lyerly HK, eds. Textbook of Surgery: *The Biological Basis of Modern Surgical Practice*, 15th Edition. Philadelphia: W. B. Saunders, 1997, pp. 815–20.
32. Paterson-Brown S, Dudley HAF. Abdominal trauma. In: Ellis BW, Paterson-Brown S, eds. *Hamilton Bailey's Emergency Surgery*, 12th Edition. Oxford: Butterworth-Heineman, 1995, pp. 474–503.
33. Burch JM, Franciose RJ, Moore EE. Trauma. In: Scwartz SI, Shires GT, Spencer FC, et al, eds. *Principles of Surgery*, 7th Edition. Vol. 1. New York: McGraw-Hill, 1999, pp, 186–8.
34. Fabian TC, Croce MA. Abdominal trauma, including indications for celiotomy. In: Mattox KL, Feliciano DV, Moore EE, eds. *Trauma*, 4th Edition. New York: McGraw-Hill, 2000, pp. 583–602.
35. Sabiston DCJ. Resection of abdominal aortic aneurysm. In: Sabiston DCJ, ed. *Atlas of General Surgery*. Philadelphia: W. B. Saunders, 1994, pp. 16–22.
36. McCann RL. Amputations. In: Sabiston DCJ, ed. *Atlas of General Surgery*. Philadelphia: W. B. Saunders, 1994, pp. 739–54.
37. Wilson, SE ed. VascularAccess: *Principles and Practice* 3rd Edition St. Louis: Mosby-Year Book, 1996.
38. Advanced Trauma Life Support for Doctors: Instructor Course Manual. Chicago: American College of Surgeons, 1997, p. 990.
39. Battistella F, Benfield J. Blunt and penetrating injuries of the chest wall, pleura, and lungs. In: Shields T, ed. *General thoracic surgery*. Philidelphia: Lippincott Williams and Wilkins, 1999.
40. Wicky S, Capasso P, Meuli R et al. Spiral CT aortography: an efficient technique for the diagnosis of traumatic aortic injury. *Eur Radiol* 8:828-33, 1998.
41. Dyer DS, Moore EE, Mestek MF et al. Can chest CT be used to exclude aortic injury? *Radiology* 213:195-202, 1999.
42. Pena A and DeVries PA. Posterior sagittal anorectoplasty: important technical considerations and new applications. *Journal of Pediatric Surgery* 17:796-811, 1982.
43. Scalea TM, Rodriguez A, Chiu WC, et al. Focused assessment with sonography for trauma: results from an international conference. *Journal of Trauma* 46:466-72, 1999.